Praise for
The Circumcision Decision: An Unbiased Guide for Parents

"In the best tradition of *Our Bodies, Ourselves,* Terkel and Greenberg have provided a beautifully balanced, evidence-based resource for parents and others thinking about the whole issue of male circumcision. The authors make clear that from a purely 'health risks and benefits' perspective, it is eminently reasonable for a parent to decide either way about circumcision. And they articulate well the various non-medical issues that can arise in making this highly-charged decision for our male children."

Judy Norsigian, founder/director of
Our Bodies Ourselves

"Outside of an often violent and condescending blogosphere, where the circumcision topic gets caught between overzealous extremist perspectives, Terkel and Greenberg provide a safe place for the hot topic to land. With grace, wisdom, and class, *The Circumcision Decision* impressively presents both sides of the story in such a balanced narrative, that some of us who have already made up our minds beforehand may now find ourselves challenged by the flip side."

Nick Shell, official daddy blogger of
Parents.com *The Dadabase*

"*The Circumcision Decision* takes an honest, balanced and human approach to the subject of circumcision to truly help a parent make a personal decision. It covers all the issues, weighs all the facts and even discusses all a parent's doubts. It's by far the best treatment of the subject I have seen yet."

Rev. Ted McIlvenna, Ph.D., president of the Institute
for Advanced Study of Human Sexuality

Praise for

The Circumcision Decision:* *An Unbiased Guide for Parents

"To circumcise or not? If you're expecting a boy, expect to be confronted with that question. For some parents, the decision is an easy one: they will...or they won't. But for those on the fence, *The Circumcision Decision* is a wonderful resource that strips away the hype and noise around this hot-button issue to focus on the cold, hard facts. Authors Susan Terkel and Lorna Greenberg present the procedure's pros and cons, risks and benefits—and the scientific evidence behind each choice—in an even-handed way. Without cheerleading or scare tactics, they provide fascinating details about circumcision's Biblical roots, chart the ebb and flow of its acceptance through history and examine the issue from every angle–religious, cultural, medical, sexual and moral. Their intent is not to sway parents one way or the other, but to provide information for parents to make their own right decision."

Norine Dworkin-McDaniel, creator of the parenting/family life blog *Don't Put Lizards In Your Ears*

"This book is an excellent resource for parents and health care providers to open the circumcision discussion."

Melissa Hines Bock, FNP, nurse practitioner and childbirth educator

The Circumcision Decision

An Unbiased Guide for Parents

Susan Terkel & Lorna Greenberg

carrot seed PUBLISHING

The intent of the authors of ***The Circumcision Decision:*** *An Unbiased Guide for Parents* has been to provide accurate information to help parents make informed judgments for themselves and their families. The authors are not medical professionals, are not providing medical advice, and suggest here, and throughout the book, that readers discuss any medical decision with their medical advisers. The authors, publisher and distributor shall not be liable or responsible for loss or damage allegedly arising from information, opinions or suggestions in this book.

info@carrotseedpublishing.com
www.carrotseedpublishing.com

book designed by Ari Terkel
illustrations by Serina Koester

ISBN 978-0-9834115-7-4

Library of Congress Cataloging-in-Publication Data
Pending

Printed in the United States of America
10 9 8 7 6 5 4 3 2 1

carrot seed PUBLISHING one east main street / hudson, oh / 44236

Acknowledgments

We have received help, advice and criticism from many sources—family, friends, rabbis, doctors, parents, and more. We especially wish to thank: Rabbi Sheldon Ezring, Dr. Alissa Greenberg, Lawrence T. Greenberg, Dr. Marjorie Greenfield, Jonathan Gross, Ph.D., Lee Haas, Peter Haas, Ph.D., Joshua Halberstam, Ph.D., Ralph L. Keeney, Ph.D., Dr. Julian Peskin, Dr. Lee Rubinstein, Rabbi Sam Stahl, Marni Terkel, Ari Terkel, and our supportive and patient spouses: Ron Greenberg and Larry Terkel.

In memory of **Pamela Morgan,**
a beloved friend whose work with the Boston Women's Collective (now known as Our Bodies Ourselves) gave Susan her perspective on health and social issues, including challenging the status quo.

CONTENTS

INTRODUCTION

Making a decision for the right reason

When you're expecting a baby, it's easy to be overwhelmed by all the choices and decisions. Physician or midwife? Home birth or hospital birth? Nurse or bottle feed? Crib or family bed? You may not even know the gender yet, but if the infant is a boy, you will face still another decision—The Circumcision Decision.

At any time in his life, a male can have a medical problem that necessitates surgical removal of his foreskin. But this book isn't about that. It's about routine neonatal circumcision, about *electing* to have an infant son circumcised sometime in the first days, weeks or months of his life. Or deciding not to have him circumcised and leaving his foreskin intact, on his penis, the way it was when he was born.

For many, and perhaps for most, parents, the decision to circumcise or not is intuitive, and doesn't arouse much internal debate. Do it. Or don't do it. According to behavioral economist and Nobel Laureate Daniel Kahneman, Ph.D., author of *Thinking, Fast and Slow*, that fast, intuitive way of making a decision is how most of us make most of our decisions. It's great for many of them, especially the hundreds of ordinary decisions we need to make every day—from which bread for our sandwich to how much time to allow to get to a dental appointment.

Thinking fast and intuitively is also a great way to respond to an emergency situation that requires a quick, decisive, intuitive reaction. But when making a decision about the body part that is the focus of the circumcision decision—knowing how important a penis is to a male and to his future partners—we think the decision deserves a slow, cognitive approach, that will involve information, reason, rationality and good use of your intellect, not just your gut feeling.

We set out to write a short book about circumcision to fill the gap between the pro-circumcision books and websites and the anti-circumcision books and websites, all of which work earnestly and often effectively, to convince you to adopt their position. We wanted to give you a balanced, accurate, and fair book to help you make a smart decision about circumcision. We also thought that the decision deserves more information than the few pages most books for expectant parents devote to the decision. And we decided that the subject was serious enough and interesting enough for us to devote more than a year of our lives to research and write it!

What we offer you is a thoughtful book that explores all sides and aspects of what is a many-faceted issue, because the first thing we learned is that circumcision is not a simple "should we or should we not?" decision. There are numerous factors and reasons to consider and explore, some of which needn't be deciding ones and others that get overlooked when they should be considered.

But most importantly, our purpose is not to persuade you to circumcise or to leave your son's foreskin intact. It is to help you make an informed, carefully considered, smart decision for your son.

Why it can be a difficult-to-make decision

Because most men in the United States are circumcised, many of us, especially those of us who are female, have never seen a man with a foreskin—an "intact" man. And many of us, including men, know very little about foreskins. For example, we learned that an adult male's foreskin measures 12 to 16 square inches and contains tens of thousands of sensitive nerve endings. We also learned that without good hygiene, a foreskin tends to harbor bacteria, and can become odorous. We learned how common it is for a foreskin to be too tight to allow for a comfortable erection or any erection at all.

We learned that many questions surround the issue of circumcision. How safe is a circumcision? Does a circumcision hurt, and does it harm an infant? Who is qualified to perform a circumcision? Should a circumciser use pain relief or a protective shield? Can an intact man still be Jewish or be Muslim? Do a circumcised man and his partner enjoy sex more or less than an intact man and his partner? What's the difference between a high and low or tight and loose circumcision? Do you have the right to decide to circumcise your son or should you let him make the decision, later? Is circumcision moral or should it be regarded as immoral, or perhaps even as mutilation? Is it important for your son to look like his father? And those are just a few of the questions to consider!

After exploring all the questions and factors to be considered, we will help you make a smart, educated, informed and rational decision about circumcising your son or leaving his foreskin intact. We'll even show you how to live with the decision you make.

Where do we stand?

As we said, many people make the circumcision decision intuitively and quickly, without much research or deliberation. Count us among the guilty! Like many parents in past decades, we never questioned circumcision, never asked about pain relief or use of protective shields. We would have done things differently if we had known then what we have learned in our research for this book. Now, one of us is pro-circumcision (pro-circ) and would make the same decision. But would have the circumcision at a different time and place and would have asked more questions about the procedure, such as about pain relief and protective shields and how to choose a circumciser. The other has become moderately anti-circumcision (anti-circ). Our different views give this book balance, since we were always alert, and called each other out whenever we detected bias.

Speaking of bias

To ensure accurate information and a fair perspective, we read every book we could find on the subject, visited Internet sites of every opinion, and interviewed clergy, ritual circumcisers, pediatricians, a urologist, obstetricians, an anesthesiologist, nurses, midwives and other professionals. We talked to men circumcised at birth and men circumcised as teens or adults—with or without their consent. We spoke to parents who regretted their decision, parents who labored over the decision, and parents who made the decision easily and with no regrets. We interviewed women whose experience allowed them to compare sex with intact and circumcised men.

A respected ethicist read the relevant chapters, as did several rabbis and a professor of religion. The coauthor of a valued decision-making book helped us with the last chapter on making a smart decision. We interviewed some gay men about circumcision and sex. Given all those interviews and input, we are now confident that we have covered all the issues you need to learn about, and covered them with a well-rounded perspective.

What we promise

The ideal time to make the decision is at least a month or two before your child is born, at a time when you are well-rested, in a good mood, have had time to learn about and think through the issues and to discuss the decision with your partner and perhaps your physician or birth-attendant. We believe that after reading this book you will be able to make a smart, rational decision. Someday, your son may challenge your decision, he may take issue with that decision, but it is likely that he will respect the care, love, and attention that went into making it.

SECTION ONE

The medical issues

CHAPTER ONE

What's a foreskin & what's a foreskin for?

A major issue in the decision to remove or keep a foreskin is whether the foreskin has a purpose, and if it does, how important is that purpose? Opinions run the gamut, from "a foreskin is a useless flap of skin" to "a foreskin is a vital part of the male anatomy."

Advocates of this second view note that every feature of the body has a purpose—even the often-dismissed appendix is thought to play a role in kidney function. The foreskin contains thousands of nerve endings and special immune-system cells, produces a natural lubricant, and protects a significant portion of a pleasure-producing organ.

Think of this chapter as an introduction to the anatomy of the foreskin and other parts of the penis. The aim is to provide information so you can make an informed decision about the medical issues involved in circumcision. Note that we said "medical issues." Sometimes a decision is based on religious beliefs or traditions, or on cultural attitudes, such as the importance of "looking like dad," or " fitting in," or other non-medical concerns. For some people, medical issues are sometimes the only ones considered. In order to make a good (for you) decision, we think you might want to start with finding out more about what you are deciding to keep or remove.

Labels

Circumcision is now such a hot issue that finding neutral terms for "cutting or keeping" is difficult. For clarity, we will refer to a penis with a foreskin as "intact" and a penis without a foreskin as "circumcised." Those who advocate circumcision will be informally called "pro-circs," opponents will be "anti-circs," or "intactavists."

We should mention the rare circumstance in which a baby seems to be born without a foreskin. The child is neither intact nor circumcised. No circumcision is needed—unless the hole for passing urine is on the underside instead of the end of the penis, in which case, corrective surgery is necessary. Again, this condition is exceedingly rare—even though some traditions say that Adam and Noah, and Mohammad are in the same elite league of being born without a foreskin.

In the beginning

The sexual organs begin to form about eight weeks after conception. The penile shaft, or penis, forms from connective tissue. The rounded end of the penis looks like an acorn. In fact, the medical term for it is glans penis, or just glans, which is Latin for acorn. The foreskin starts to form toward the end of the first trimester of pregnancy. It forms out of tissue growing on the outside of the penis. This tissue grows so quickly that it folds over into a flap that covers the glans. It's called a foreskin because it is at the fore, or the front, of the penis. Another name is prepuce.

Nature's sleeve: a protector

Imagine dressing your infant son in a hoodie. It's a chilly day and you pull the sleeves over his hands so the fleece lining will protect them. You gently pull each hand through the stretchy, ribbed end of the sleeve. You can scrunch the sleeves up, onto his wrists. You can fold the sleeves back over his wrists. You can even push the sleeves up and down. Foreskins are a bit like sleeves. They start about halfway down the penile shaft. Instead of fleece, foreskins have a moist tissue lining. At its end, the foreskin has a ribbed, stretchy opening—called a meatus.

Like a sleeve, a foreskin can slide up and down the round end of the penis (the glans). The foreskin can be pulled backward, which exposes its lining. It can also be scrunched up above the glans. And finally, an erect penis pushes the glans out through the meatus.

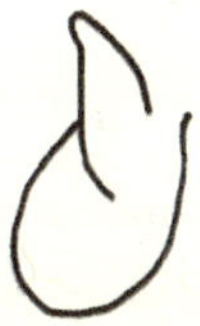

UNCIRCUMCISED

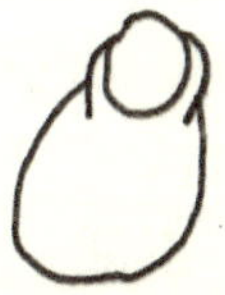

CIRCUMCISED

The multi-tasking foreskin

The foreskin has an important role in protecting the penis. The outer layer of the foreskin is like the skin on the penis. The mucosal inner layer is moist tissue that produces an oily substance (sebum). These two tissue layers are similar to those of the eyelid—a top layer of skin, and a moisture-producing inner layer.

When sebum combines with shed skin cells, it forms a natural emollient called smegma—from a Greek word for soap. If smegma is allowed to collect under the foreskin and mix with moisture and bacteria and become stale, it can develop an unpleasant odor—not in the least like Dove or Dial. The irony is that this lubricant can then be a turnoff to sex rather than an enhancement. Careful washing is usually enough to avoid the odor problem. With the help of smegma, the foreskin can glide back over the glans and the penis. And the penis can glide through the foreskin.

Among its other functions, the foreskin contains thousands of nerve cells that make it exceedingly sensitive to touch. It also contains thousands of immune-system cells that fight infection and inflammation. Here's another irony: while these cells fight some infections, they may allow HIV and other viruses to bind to them and enter the body, multiply and cause havoc.

Separation issues

When the foreskin first develops, it is fused to the glans by a thin tissue layer or membrane, called the synechia. The synechia dissolves over time—usually a short time. In 10 percent of male infants, it has dissolved by birth. For most boys, it dissolves before they begin elementary school. About 10 percent of boys still have a foreskin attached, at least partially, by adolescence. In a few cases, a circumcision is needed. If the synechia remains attached, it can make an erection painful or even impossible.

Most males can loosen their foreskins themselves with gentle massage and stretching, which often occurs when a boy "plays with himself," a process that should take place in private, of course. If it hasn't separated or is only partially separated, a boy's pediatrician can help with suggestions to loosen it. However, because the synechia is tissue with blood flowing through it, it should never be pulled off the glans. That can cause bleeding and infection. This is the reason we caution you to never forcibly pull the foreskin off the glans.

Once the foreskin is no longer fused to the glans, it can be pulled back for cleaning. And pulled back and forth for pleasure, for masturbation, foreplay, and intercourse.

Keeping the foreskin in place

A small connective tissue called a frenulum, located on the underside of the penis, holds the foreskin over the glans. When the foreskin folds over or gets scrunched behind the glans, the frenulum helps to bring it back in place.

Some men say their frenulum is sensitive to touch and this may be a reason not to remove it in a circumcision. It's more likely, however, that the rich supply of nerves under the frenulum is responsible for that sensitivity.

Getting an erection

Underneath the skin of the penis, but not in the foreskin, is spongy tissue that fills with blood during an erection. Erections often occur during the REM sleep cycle. And they occur during masturbation, foreplay, and sometimes during thoughts about sex.

QUESTION: Where does the foreskin go during an erection?

ANSWER: It slides back, scrunches up, or folds over.

A few words about foreskin size

Like penises, foreskins vary in size. They range from 12 to 16 square inches on an adult man (only a square inch or so on an infant). They also vary in proportion to the rest of the penis. Some cover half or more of the penis; others cover a third or less—of a flaccid (non-erect) penis, that is.

Many—or most (we haven't conducted a reliable survey for this fact and don't really trust the Internet) foreskins end beyond the tip of the glans, giving the penis the illusion of extra length. Others end at the tip of the glans and a few end before the tip, leaving part of the glans exposed.

When appearances count

Intact and circumcised penises look quite different when they are flaccid. Foreskins make the intact penis resemble a banana. A circumcised penis, with an exposed glans and a corona (a raised rim around the base of the glans) looks more like an acorn attached to a big tube.

Shape isn't the only difference. Because the foreskin usually covers, protects and moistens the glans, the skin on that glans appears shiny and lighter in skin tone. Without a protective foreskin, the glans of a circumcised penis is more exposed to abrasion and dryness. Its skin is probably tougher and less vulnerable to scratches. The skin may be desensitized and this may reduce sexual pleasure. (But talking about sex is jumping ahead. Here we are focusing on the medical issues.)

Up close, the foreskin may be folded back over the penis, exposing its moist lining. Or the foreskin may be bunched behind the corona. Or the foreskin may cover just some of the glans.

The real issue: a useless flap of skin, or not?

We believe the foreskin is not a useless flap of skin—nor is this a dull topic. So now, let's tackle the real issue. What's a foreskin for? Note that we will present a number of plausible (and debatable) theories.

The foreskin protects the glans from waste

One theory is that the purpose of a foreskin is to protect the male sexual organ in the womb. Since it covers the glans, it protects both the glans and its opening to the urethra (the tube that will eventually carry urine and semen out of the body) from exposure to fecal matter and other detritus circulating in the amniotic fluid. The problem with this theory is that it fails to explain why 10 percent of newborns have retractable foreskins, therefore lacking the protection. Does this fact undermine the theory? Or is it a reminder that there are no perfect answers in an imperfect world?

Foreskins protect the glans from abrasion and from possible infection

The foreskin shields the skin on the glans from scratches and bruises, and moisturizes it. Thus, some theorists believe the foreskin has an evolutionary basis. Before loincloths, underwear and jock straps, the foreskin protected the glans from getting scratched or injured by underbrush or other natural hazards. In addition, the lubrication and sensitivity it provided may have enabled early humans to have intercourse more easily and quickly—and thus at less risk of attack from prowling animals.

The foreskin has protective value against infection. It has a sphincter function to keep out infectious material and a rich blood supply to fight contaminants.

Foreskins enhance sex

With its tens of thousands of sensitive and sensual nerve endings (meaning that their neurons easily send sexual messages to the brain), its ability to glide back and forth over the penis, especially over the sensitive glans, the most significant role for the foreskin may be for sex and therefore, also, for reproduction.

First, prior to sex, the gliding movement of a foreskin can trigger sexual desire and send the brain a signal to produce hormones that will send blood to create an erection. The gliding movement over the end of the penis increases sensitivity and adds to sexual pleasure for both the man and his partner. Thus, the foreskin may enhance sex, although some theorists have stated that this enhancement may make a guy too lustful, too quick to ejaculate, or too preoccupied with sex to do other important things in his life—which may provide reasons to justify removal of foreskins.

Like some other organs and tissues of the body, a foreskin can be removed. And most of the time, for most males, removing it won't dramatically change their lives (even if some men on the Internet claim that it does). Still, what we hope you have learned is that while foreskins can be removed, and occasionally need to be removed for medical reasons (information about this in Chapter 3), the foreskin is not a *totally* useless flap of skin—but it is also not essential (especially after the child is born). Still, many people throughout the world consider those 12 to 16 square inches of tissue worth keeping.

DIRECTIONS

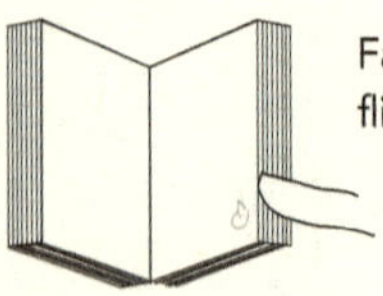

Fan the pages then flip the corners.

CHAPTER TWO

What's a circumcision?

In this chapter we will tell you all you need to know about the mechanics of circumcision. We left out most medical jargon, but included all the essential information, and a little advice.

The Basics

A circumcision is a procedure to remove the foreskin (or prepuce) from a penis. In earlier times, only the tip of the foreskin was removed. In most infant circumcision today, nearly all the foreskin is removed—that is, the outer layer, the inner layer and the frenulum. [A frenulum—from the Latin word meaning "small bridle"—is an elastic band of tissue that restricts the movements of a body part. The body has other frenula, such as tissues under the tongue and inside the lips.]

How much of the foreskin is removed, where the scar from the cut will lie on the penile shaft, and how much of the inner layer is left all depend on the size and shape of the penis and foreskin, the circumciser's technique, and the method used. It is hard to imagine how a circumciser determines the amount of skin to leave, since it is impossible to know the length of the future adult's erect penis. But doctors and trained circumcisers who have performed many circumcisions say it is a simple decision and procedure, and for them, it probably is.

A VISUAL AID

The following is an animated illustration of a circumcision which uses a popular shield to protect the glans. Pain relief would be administered before the procedure.

THIS IS A SURGICAL PROCEDURE, VIEWING IT MAY BE INNAPROPRIATE FOR SOME

Pain relief

Before we describe the circumcision procedure, we need to pause to talk about the important topic of pain relief. For centuries, circumcisers claimed that newborns did not feel pain, that their brains and nervous systems were too immature to register pain. Some circumcisers (and parents) disagreed, but the belief persisted. Then, in 1987, Harvard Medical School-Boston Children's Hospital completed a landmark study of pain responses in newborns. The results provided solid evidence that newborns, in fact, do feel pain, and that their pain pathways are well-developed by birth. In that study and later ones, researchers tracked changes in infants' heart rates and rhythm, blood pressure and oxygen levels, breathing, levels of stress hormones, crying, responses to caregivers, sleep patterns, facial expressions and other behaviors. All showed that circumcision is extremely painful and babies register the pain. If some don't cry, they may be in shock. If some seem to sleep through the procedure, they may have retreated into a semi-comatose state. Although some circumcisers still insist pain relief is not necessary, the evidence that infants do feel pain is clear and definitive. Since pain relief is safe and available, why should an infant suffer?

Steps to reduce pain

Most importantly, the parents should select a circumciser who is able and ready to provide effective pain relief. (The word infant comes from the Latin, *infans*, which means without a voice, or unable to speak. You need to act as the voice for your child.) Traditional circumcisers and nurse-midwives and others can use topical medications that may reduce pain, and may also use traditional methods of soothing the infant—such as a quiet, calm setting with soft music or a tape of intrauterine sounds, swaddling, the comfort of a parent's voice and touch. Sucking on a gloved finger, a pacifier or a piece of gauze dipped in a sugar solution (24 percent sucrose) may also help. Researchers think the sweet taste stimulates opiate pathways in the brain (which may be why the drops of sweet wine traditional circumcisers give infants sometimes seem to calm them). But in the face of the severe pain of circumcision—especially when the foreskin is torn from the glans, or when the foreskin layers are clamped and cut away, all on a very sensitive body part—these techniques are clearly insufficient.

The American Academy of Pediatrics states that circumcision is an invasive, painful procedure and that failure to provide pain control is *unethical.* They recommend that infants be given pain control during and after circumcision.

Researchers report these possible reasons for some circumcisers' failure to offer pain relief: some claim that their skill and speed make it unnecessary, some persist in the belief that babies do not feel pain, some question the value of anesthetics, some are reluctant to ask parents for the necessary consent, some are disinterested or lack training in pain control. You may hear a circumciser claim that in skilled hands, the procedure is quick and painless. We think this is a signal to find another circumciser.

While general anesthesia is risky for infants, and is not used in infant circumcisions, there are safe, effective pain-relief options to discuss with your doctor.

Topical pain relief

A prescription topical cream (EMLA: a mixture of local anesthetics) can provide slight to moderate relief. It is spread over the lower half of the penis an hour or two before the procedure, to numb the skin. It is easy to use, but at a busy facility, the preparation time may be a problem. Nor does the cream penetrate deeply enough to fully control intense pain. In addition, some infants may be sensitive to an ingredient in the cream.

Injected pain relief

More effective choices include the dorsal penile nerve block (DPNB) and the ring block. In DPNB, two deep injections of Lidocaine are given at the base of the penis. This reduces the pain significantly. For a ring block, Lidocaine is injected under the skin, in a ring around the penile shaft, midway down from the tip. The ring block is thought to be the most consistently effective measure for pain relief. If an infant seems in pain after the circumcision, he may be given infant Tylenol.

The Circumcision

In a routine newborn circumcision in a hospital, medical facility or birthing center, the infant may be strapped onto a molded plastic board (called a "Circumstraint"). In some facilities the board is padded and warmed, or an adjustable circumcision chair is used, which holds the infant in a more comfortable position. These are nice, but not essential, improvements. In a home circumcision, the infant may be strapped to a board or held by a parent, relative or family friend. Velcro straps may be wrapped around his legs, and often his arms too, so they won't jostle the circumciser.

Since the infant has been curled up in the womb through pregnancy, stretching out his limbs may start him crying. Leaving his arms free—so he can suck his fingers or hold a parent's finger—may help.

The first step in a circumcision is to separate the foreskin from the glans, since it is stuck onto the glans in 90 percent of newborns. The separation is usually done with a long metal probe. Next, most circumcisers make a small vertical cut (a dorsal slit) in the foreskin. This allows the circumciser to inspect the glans to make sure it is properly formed. If there is any abnormality, such as the opening to allow urine to exit is not at the end of the glans but on the lower surface, the circumcision may not be completed. That's because the foreskin may be needed for a skin graft to correct the problem surgically.

In the next step, the circumciser prepares to cut off the foreskin. Most circumcisers use a clamp, such as the Gomco or Mogen clamp, to protect the glans from an accidental cut and to reduce bleeding by crushing the foreskin tissue. The circumciser sets the clamp in place, and presses on the handle to cut off the foreskin's blood supply. After a few minutes, the foreskin is cut off.

If the Plastibell device is used instead of a clamp, there is no cutting except for the dorsal slit. The foreskin is stretched over a plastic bell, a cord is tied around it to crush it and stop the blood supply. The foreskin tissue dies and falls off by itself, usually in about a week.

The technique a circumciser chooses will depend on his or her training. Sometimes it is determined by the infant's anatomy, since some infants have layers of fat surrounding the area where the penis begins. The procedure is over quickly—sometimes in a few minutes, and nearly always in less than 20 minutes. The time depends on the circumciser's skill and experience, and the technique.

An infant's skin layers are very thin and heal quickly, so there is no need for stitches. The circumcised penis is dressed in sterile gauze. Within days or a week or so, the circumcision will have completely healed. Sometimes there is some extra bleeding that can be treated by pressure, and sometimes the cut develops a minor infection that can be treated with a topical antibiotic. Once the procedure is over, if the infant's diapers are changed regularly, all will be well. (In Chapter 4, however, we will describe what can go wrong.)

Who performs circumcisions?

In the U.S., all physicians are licensed to perform newborn circumcisions. Many are specifically trained to do circumcision—obstetricians who deliver babies, pediatricians, family doctors, surgeons and urologists. Certified nurse-midwives may also train to perform newborn circumcisions.

Because circumcision is a religious rite for Jews and Muslims, within those religious groups some individuals learn to perform circumcisions and to recite the prayers and conduct the rituals that accompany a circumcision. A traditional Jewish circumciser is called a mohel, or a mohelot for a female. Many learned how to perform circumcisions from their fathers. (And were often required to perform their first circumcision on their own newborn son.) Today, the Union for Reform Judaism (URJ) sponsors a program to train and license mohels, as does the American Board of Ritual Circumcision. Hebrew Union College of New York certifies mohels who have trained in circumcision techniques and traditions. Some Jewish doctors learn the prayers and the rituals and become physician/mohels (our preferred choice—for a mohel).

In Islam, circumcision is believed to enhance cleanliness and purity, and serves as an introduction to the Islamic faith and as a sign of belonging to the Muslim community. Unlike Jewish circumcision, there is no fixed age or set procedure. The timing and the rituals vary by culture or community. Thus, in some Islamic communities, circumcision is performed on the seventh day after birth, while in others it is performed during childhood, or at puberty. Some Muslim boys are circumcised after they have learned to recite the entire Qur'an. The Muslim ceremony is often a festive one, with music, special food and celebration.

In earlier times, the Muslim circumciser was a member of the community who had learned the procedure through watching and helping previous generations of circumcisers. Now, traditional circumcisions are less common, and many Muslim families are choosing to have their sons circumcised at birth, by a doctor, at a hospital or a medical clinic. In Muslim societies that circumcise boys during childhood or puberty, a licensed circumcising surgeon may conduct the procedure at a home or in a hospital or clinic.

When

Most circumcisions are performed on infants who are only a day or two old. That's because today, most mothers and their infants are discharged from the hospital that quickly. And often, especially for the birth of a first child, mothers are eager to pick up the infant and go home.

Jewish circumcisions traditionally take place on the eighth day of the infant's life. There are benefits from this tradition. First, it allows time for the infant's doctor to know that the infant is healthy enough for a circumcision. Second it gives the mother and infant a chance to bond, and to establish a feeding routine—especially helpful if the mother is nursing her infant. By the beginning of the second week of life, the infant and his mother have had a chance to recover from the birth trauma. Yet he still has the high levels of stress hormones, such as adrenaline, cortisol, and endorphins, that helped him through the birth trauma and which can now help him through the trauma of circumcision.

And how much

Most major medical insurers cover newborns' circumcisions. About thirty state Medicaid plans will also cover them. However, if you postpone circumcision, few insurers and almost no Medicaid plans will pay for an elective circumcision. They will, however, pay for a circumcision to treat a medical condition, such as phimosis or recurring urinary tract infections.

The cost differences between a newborn's circumcision and one for a baby a few months older can be considerable—even thousands of dollars. The major reason for the difference is that newborns don't receive general anesthesia and don't require sutures, whereas boys do. Complications—bleeding and infection—are more common for older children.

A newborn's routine hospital circumcision may cost several hundred dollars or less. A religious circumcision, at home or elsewhere, may cost a few hundred to a thousand dollars more (especially if you factor in food trays, beverages and desserts). The cost will still be less than the cost of a medical circumcision for an older child, which currently costs between $2,500 and $4,000. It may be more if you wait several years. And, insurance coverage is uncertain. If your son is older than two or three months, or weighs fifteen pounds or more, his foreskin will have grown thicker and stitches may be necessary. There is greater risk of bleeding and other complications, and healing will take longer.

Circumcisions for men

Adult men are most often circumcised in hospitals, with general anesthesia. A new commercial circumcision technique, called the PrePex, has been developed for adults who choose to have an elective circumcision, perhaps for a religious reason or as a protective health measure. Its developers promote it especially for use in areas of Africa where there is a high rate of HIV infection, to protect men from contracting the virus from female sex partners. It is described as inexpensive, simple to use, causing no pain or bleeding, requiring no stitches, and there is no risk of accidental cuts. It can only be used on males whose foreskin has separated from the glans. It is FDA-approved, but not yet available in the U.S.

The PrePex device is similar to the Plastibell and the Tara Klamp. Plastic rings are applied to the foreskin to cut off its blood supply, thus forcing it to die. About a week later, the rings and the foreskin are cut off. A PrePex circumcision does not fulfill the Jewish circumcision requirement of some bleeding, but it can be accompanied by pricking the penis for a token amount of blood.

Different cuts for different circs

In ancient times, only the tip of the foreskin—that part that normally extends past the end of the glans—was removed. Modern circumcisions remove all or most of the foreskin. Orthodox Jewish circumcisions require the removal of the foreskin with just one cut.

Some circumcisions leave extra skin on the penis that can bunch up behind the glans or hang over the glans a little when the penis is flaccid. This extra skin can also move up and down the penile shaft, even when the penis is erect. Such circumcisions are "loose" circumcisions. We have been told that Israeli circumcisions tend to be loose while tight circumcisions are more common elsewhere, perhaps because of the specific circumcision devices used. Some circumcision scars are high on the penile shaft, others are lower. Some circumcisers choose to leave a small amount of foreskin on the penis.

Experience counts

We encourage you to find a circumciser who has been well trained and has a lot of experience. Among doctors—obstetricians, pediatricians, urologists and physician/mohels generally have had the most experience in circumcising. While non-physician mohels may have years of experience, they cannot provide injectable pain relief.

A circumciser who has performed hundreds or even thousands of circumcisions is less likely to botch a circumcision by accidentally cutting into the glans, and is more likely to recognize when a penis should not be circumcised.

Occasionally, the area where the foreskin was cut may bleed a little or develop a minor infection or be sensitive. Most infants recover quickly. Rarely, some foreskin tissue may be left, and it may adhere to the glans and need to be removed. Some other—usually minor—problem may need to be corrected in a simple medical procedure. The next chapter discusses more significant problems. While most occur rarely, they are the stories that lead some parents to choose not to circumcise their infant!

Circumcision for healthy babies, only

Routine newborn circumcision is elective surgery. Even by religious law, it is mandated only for healthy babies. Thus, if an infant is premature or unstable, if his birth weight is too low (under 5 pounds), if there is any illness or abnormality, the circumcision should be postponed. If there is any reason to question the health of the infant, perhaps the child should not be circumcised.

If there is reason to suspect a familial bleeding disorder, such as hemophilia, postpone the circumcision or leave the child intact. If a parent, grandparent, sibling, aunt or uncle has had excessive bleeding or other complications after a minor procedure, consult a doctor. The infant may need to be tested for a bleeding disorder before planning a circumcision.

Finally, if there is a malformation or anomaly of the penis, the circumcision should be postponed as the foreskin may be needed for skin grafting in a procedure to correct the condition.

In conclusion

Ah, what conclusions to draw from all this? First, circumcision is a medical procedure, and therefore, we believe, should be performed by a medically trained circumciser. This is our opinion. We do understand that some people feel it is important to use a traditional circumciser and that is their choice.

Second, only a healthy infant who weighs at least 5 pounds and has no family history of excessive bleeding, should be circumcised.

Third, there is abundant, well-documented evidence that infants do feel pain. Thus, we believe infants should be provided with effective pain relief.

And last, as stated earlier, we believe that the best person to perform your son's circumcision is a well-trained physician (or physician/mohel) who has a good deal of circumcision experience.

Circumcision has been performed successfully throughout history, long before antibiotics, even long before surgical instruments were invented. Still, it is a medical procedure. So, if you decide to have your newborn circumcised, find an experienced circumciser, who will provide effective pain relief and who gives you a sense of confidence that everything is likely to go well. We know that many mohels have performed many circumcisions—successfully. But we feel a physicians' (or a physician/mohel's) ability to offer more effective pain relief, greater and broader medical knowledge and training and ability to handle unexpected complications are invaluable assets.

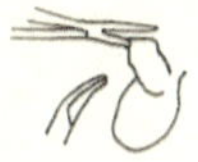

ADDENDUM:

What happens to all those foreskins?

In early Judaism, and in other early cultures, the severed foreskin was thought to have mystical powers and was often buried. Later—when most Jews no longer lived so close to the land—mohels brought parents a bowl of sand or soil in which to place the foreskin to save it. Some traditional Jews still follow this practice. In a newer tradition, more popular in Israel, parents bury the foreskin under a sapling. When the boy marries, branches from that sapling are used for the wedding canopy.

Other ancient cultures followed a variety of rituals: some burned the foreskins, some dried and saved them, hoping they would ensure another male infant. In some cultures, they were fed to domestic animals; in others they were dried, mixed with food, and fed back to the circumcised boy so that his body would be complete if resurrected. In some Muslim cultures, the foreskin was made into a salve, "Oil of Man," which was used to aid healing—including healing the circumcision wound.

Today, in hospital circumcisions, the foreskin is usually disposed of with other medical wastes. However, in recent decades, scientists have learned that this small, limp sac of tissue has significant properties and considerable commercial value. Biotechnology researchers are able to culture human skin tissue from fibroblasts, which are cells of the foreskin. The fibroblasts are used to grow bio-engineered skin, which is used for burn victims, to cover diabetic ulcers, to produce interferonbased drugs, and to make cosmetic products, including wrinkle creams. Consequently, some private hospitals and birthing centers sell foreskins to bio-medical research laboratories, and also to cosmetics companies. David Gollaher, in his book, *Circumcision,* states that one boy's foreskin can yield 250,000 square feet of a skin replacement product called LSEs, (living skin equivalents), an amount about equal to the size of a football field. Since the product can be sold for $3,000 dollars a square foot, and well over a million foreskins are circumcised in the United States each year, this is big business.

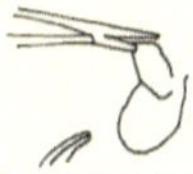

CHAPTER THREE

Why circumcise?
Potential benefits/possible risks

In an earlier chapter, we made a case for the usefulness of the foreskin. But—while it may provide benefits—the foreskin, like any other body part, is subject to medical problems. Some problems arise out of neglect, such as neglecting to keep the foreskin clean enough, which can lead to infections or body odor.

Some problems develop from a physical condition, such as a foreskin that is too tight or has failed to separate off the glans. And sometimes the problem isn't caused by the foreskin, but the foreskin still gets the rap—such as when it is blamed for causing penile cancer, which is more likely to be caused by frequent sex with many different partners (especially starting at an early age), by smoking, or by a serious lack of hygiene over a long period.

And many people, including doctors, believe removing the foreskin will help to prevent potential problems. Circumcisions performed at a later age are usually treatment for an existing (not potential) medical problem.

However, many of the problems blamed on foreskins, such as foul odors and infections, are easy to prevent and easy to treat. Since that is the case, many parents choose to leave their son's foreskin intact. And

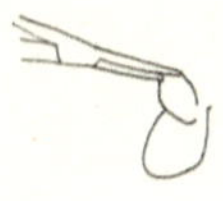

they are willing to gamble on the risks of more serious issues, such as sexually transmitted diseases (STDs), including HIV, for reasons you will read about in this chapter.

Judging the medical issues requires interpreting statistics accurately and being as unbiased as possible. We are often troubled by the biased, and sometimes vitriolic, presentations we see on many circumcision websites. Their goal seems to be to convince people to adopt their views about circumcision, rather than to educate their readers. What follows in this chapter—and the rest of the book—is as unbiased a presentation as possible. As we sit on different sides of the issue, we therefore don't allow each other to rationalize or draw irrational conclusions. Our purpose is not to persuade you to take a side, but rather to provide full information about the medical issues, the cultural and moral issues, the sexual and human issues; and to present the opposing arguments so you will be able to make your own intelligent, rational, and carefully thought-out decision for your son.

Prevention versus treatment

Our first, and an important, point is that the decision to circumcise a newborn for potential medical benefits is *elective.* That is, it is a choice based on the belief—or hope—that the circumcision will provide future health advantages or benefits, or prevent certain medical problems. In contrast, an existing medical condition may *require* a circumcision to treat or cure it. Medically necessary circumcisions are not the focus here. This book is about "routine neonatal circumcision"—that is, *elective* circumcision of a newborn male.

Example of circumcision used to prevent a problem
Remove a newborn's foreskin and his risk of contracting some sexually transmitted diseases may be reduced. Remove the infant's foreskin and the adult male will not have a foreskin too tight to allow an erection.

Example of circumcision as a treatment for a problem
If a foreskin is too tight to allow an erection, it may need to be removed.

Hygiene and health

Many foreskin problems can be prevented with two simple habits, the HH Habits. The first is "Hands Off!" and the second is "Hygiene."

"Hands Off" means never force a foreskin off a glans (or tear the connecting tissue) while the foreskin is still attached—either by synechia or because the foreskin is too tight. Never! It is likely to cause pain and bleeding, and perhaps an infection. This is a simple rule, but extraordinarily important.

"Hygiene." Old-fashioned, simple soap-and-water hygiene can prevent many of the problems associated with foreskins. You will need to gently wash the genitals for your infant and young son. And you will need to teach him to do it himself.

One basic reason for keeping the foreskin clean is to prevent the mucus produced in the lining from acquiring a foul odor. Good

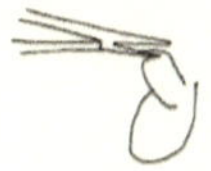

hygiene also helps to prevent bacterial infections, including urinary tract infections (UTIs) that are often cited as a reason to circumcise. Good hygiene keeps the foreskin and the glans from becoming infected or inflamed. It may reduce the risk of penile cancer, as some studies seem to indicate that regions with poor sanitation have higher rates of the disease. More about that later. Now we are emphasizing the importance of cleanliness.

Simplifying life

Many parents choose to have their son's foreskins removed because they think that will make hygiene easier. In the past, the U.S. military recommended circumcision for servicemen because hygiene with a foreskin is slightly trickier when sanitary conditions and clean water supplies are unreliable, and clean penises are healthier. Perhaps a reason slightly more intact males develop UTIs is that they don't know how to keep the penis clean—or the process seems like a hassle. Infants who get UTIs often get them during the first year, when they are in diapers. So changing diapers frequently, especially when soiled with feces, is important.

Penis hygiene is an essential habit for your son to learn. Most of us usually can rely on clean water and indoor plumbing—with occasional exceptions for hurricanes, tornadoes, power failures, earthquakes and other disasters. But there can be times—such as on long camping trips, while performing humanitarian work or military service in some areas of the world—when hygiene could be a challenge for your son. And that's when a foreskin could cause a medical problem.

Foreskin separation problem

As the male fetus develops, or after birth, or during childhood or sometimes not until adolescence, the foreskin naturally separates from the glans. In about 1 in 10 infants, the foreskin has separated by birth; but by adolescence, 1 in 10 boys will still have a foreskin that is partially or completely attached to the glans. And, this attachment can make an erection painful or impossible and make hygiene more difficult. Most boys can loosen an attached foreskin with gentle massage and gentle stretching. A pediatrician can give advice here. (Remember, a parent or caregiver should never force the separation of a foreskin from the glans.) If that doesn't work, surgery—perhaps a circumcision—may be needed. But for nearly all boys—especially those allowed to "play with themselves"— the foreskin and glans will separate without intervention.

Too tight problem

Either the entire foreskin or just its opening (meatus) can be too tight to allow the foreskin to move off the glans or allow the glans to move through the opening during an erection. This condition of being not stretchy enough is called phimosis. About 10 percent of intact children under age three will have phimosis, and about 1 percent of adult males will. For some children, phimosis may correct itself. For others, and for adults, a medical circumcision may be needed.

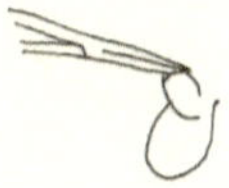

Stuck in the groove

While we wish to avoid dramatic stories that can lead you to make an irrational circumcision decision, we do need to mention an uncommon medical condition called paraphimosis, which is when a tight foreskin gets stuck in the groove above the glans, or the glans becomes swollen and the foreskin cannot retract over it. Tight foreskins stuck in grooves act like rubber bands, cutting off the supply of blood to the glans and causing swelling and, sometimes, tissue damage or tissue death. It is not unusual to see this condition in nursing homes, where men with dementia may forget to pull their foreskins back over the glans after urinating. These men may also forget to clean under the foreskin and thus suffer more UTIs. Paraphimosis may then require a circumcision. On balance, fear of paraphimosis should not be a reason to circumcise a newborn. The condition is not common and improved circumcision techniques for adult men will make the procedure less daunting.

Irritated, inflamed and infected

Sometimes the foreskin or the glans, or both, get scratched or inflamed, especially when dirt and sand get under the foreskin and irritate the lining and the glans. These problems may also be caused by a trauma, such as getting hit in the groin by a baseball, or by rough sex. And they can occur when a foreskin is forced off the glans. Here are the medical names for these conditions:

Posthitis: foreskin is irritated, inflamed or infected
Balanitis: glans is irritated, inflamed or infected
Balanoposthitis: both the foreskin and glans are irritated, inflamed or infected

Now here's the good news: except during times of war, as when troops were stationed in the deserts of Northern Africa during World War II, and other times when hygiene is difficult, posthitis, balanitis and especially balanoposthitis are exceedingly rare. More good news: these conditions can usually be treated, although a circumcision may be needed if the condition is severe or recurs.

Blame it on the foreskin

Foreskins are sometimes blamed for a number of medical infections. And in many instances, they deserve blame since having a foreskin will put a male at greater risk. However, practicing good hygiene, as well as using condoms consistently, can prevent many of the infections.

Urinary Tract Infections (UTIs)

A number of studies indicate that intact male infants are 10 times more likely to get an infection in the tube that transports urine out of the penis (and later transports semen out) than are circumcised boys. As many as half of the boys who get a urinary tract infection will get another one, and repeated infections may become a serious medical issue. But, although an intact male is at greater risk, he is not necessarily at much of a risk. That's because only 3 out of 100 intact male infants are likely to get a urinary infection in the first year of life, which means that 97 out of 100 won't get one. And many of the infections can be prevented by changing diapers frequently and practicing good hygiene. Moreover, most urinary tract infections are easy to treat.

Since our aim is to present a balanced picture, we do warn that a recurring infection or infections that are left untreated can cause serious medical problems, including kidney infections, kidney failure, brain damage, or even death. Also, while urinary tract infections are far more prevalent in girls, who get them 10 times as often as boys, when boys do get a UTI, it is more likely to lead to a kidney infection.

UTIs generally cause a fever, and sometimes a strong odor, both of which should alert you to take your son to his pediatrician, who can prescribe treatment. And while we know many of us take antibiotics too frequently, fever in an infant may need to be treated. Your doctor should make this decision. To sum up here, UTIs are uncommon—especially if hygiene is good—and usually treatable. So fear of these infections need not carry great weight in your consideration of circumcision.

Cancer of the penis

For a good many years, foreskins were blamed for a higher incidence of cancer of the penis. We now know that other factors—smoking, poor hygiene, and promiscuous sex that puts the male at risk of contracting human papilloma virus (HPV), the most common sexually transmitted virus in the United States—are the ones that actually increase a man's risk of penile cancer.

The vast majority of cancers of the penis occur in men who are older, over age 60. It may be optimistic, but it may also be likely that a male infant born today will, 60 years from now, be living in a world where cancer of the penis is preventable by vaccination or is curable.

Also, current statistics suggest that most cases of penile cancer are in intact men (1 in 400 to 600 intact men will get cancer of the penis compared to 1 in 500,000 to 18 million circumcised men, depending on the country and the specific study). Given the known factors that increase the risk of penile cancer (to repeat: age, smoking, poor hygiene, promiscuous sex), and the real possibility that there may be a means of prevention or cure by the time your son is at risk, penile cancer need not be a compelling reason to circumcise your son, despite what some physicians may tell you.

Sexually transmitted diseases and infections (STD, STIs)

Other medical conditions blamed on the foreskin include a number of sexual transmitted diseases, including syphilis, gonorrhea, genital herpes; and sexually transmitted infections, including human papilloma virus, (HPV). HPV is very common, and is a primary cause of cervical cancer. There is now an effective vaccine to protect against some strains of this virus. While only women are at risk for cervical cancer, the vaccine is often recommended for girls, women and boys and young men, to prevent transmission of the virus.

The medical issue that gets the most press in connection with circumcision is the HIV/AIDS epidemic in Africa. There, studies seem to indicate that special cells in the lining of the foreskin, cells that normally deter other infections, provide a portal for infecting a male with HIV that can lead to AIDS. Some researchers find the statistical evidence conclusive and support the recent campaign in some African countries to circumcise adult men, especially men with HIV-positive female partners. It is believed that circumcision can dramatically reduce their risk of being infected with HIV by as much as 60 percent. Again, as with penile cancer, the issue may not be a factor in your decision if you live in a culture, such as the U.S., where HIV/AIDS tends to be acquired through needle-sharing and through unprotected homosexual intercourse. And, as with penile cancer, researchers may develop a preventive vaccine (as there now is for some types of HPV) or an effective treatment by the time your son grows up. Unlike the situation with penile cancer, where only infant circumcision appears to provide protection, circumcision for adults may be protective. We do wish to point out that condoms will afford much of the same protection.

Our say

To sum up, a foreskin (like any body part) can cause a medical problem—one that can produce pain and can lead to a more serious problem. These problems can sometimes be prevented or treated easily. Importantly, the problems tend to be rare for people practicing good hygiene and other good habits—including not smoking and practicing safe sex. This puts less responsibility on the foreskin and more on the individual's good habits and healthy lifestyle.

Given the organ in question, it seems unfair to put foreskins in the category of wisdom teeth, which routinely are removed to prevent medical problems. Some of the blame heaped on the foreskin has been over-stated or overly dramatized—and some is just wrong. Still, foreskins can cause a medical problem, but as we learn in the next few chapters, so can circumcisions. In fact, what we will learn is that the statistics tend to be similar—the percentage of intact boys who will get a minor, treatable, urinary infection in their first year of life will be about the same as the percentage of circumcised boys who will get a minor, treatable complication from the circumcision procedure. Thus, we feel, the gamble is yours—and either way it isn't much of a gamble when you give your son healthy habits, especially good hygiene and medical attention when a problem does arise.

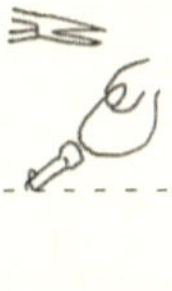

CHAPTER FOUR

Avoiding problems

One of the most common reasons parents choose not to circumcise their newborns is fear of what might go wrong during or after the circumcision. Often, they've heard a tragic story about a baby who hemorrhaged and died, or who developed a life-threatening infection. Or they've heard of a botched circumcision, especially one in which part or all of the glans was cut off.

These dramatic stories affect us and scare us because they are true. Also because they affected an innocent infant who didn't really *need* the circumcision but whose parents *chose* to have him circumcised.

Rationally, we know that the probability of a terrible outcome is miniscule. That any serious complications occur, at all, however, is proof that they might happen. And that is enough to convince some parents not to put their infant son at risk—at all.

The stories of "circumcisions gone wrong" affect a parent's decision-making in two ways. First, the stories allow emotions to take the place of sensible thinking and objectivity. Secondly, if a person is averse to risk-taking (and parenthood seems to foster risk-aversion), the fact that something awful has *ever* happened allows that person to adopt a position without thinking about it from a reasonable perspective, such as evaluating the actual risk level.

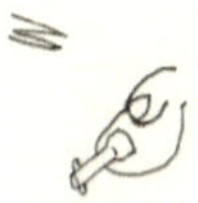

Because dramatic stories can be given too much importance, we won't focus on them. Besides, you can find them on numerous websites aimed at persuading you to adopt an anti-circumcision position. However, we will tell you what might possibly go wrong during or after a circumcision—in part, to support our advice to use a licensed, experienced circumciser. Also, we think that if we discuss the actual risks objectively, with a minimum of drama, we can help you make an intelligent, thought-out decision.

Gaining perspective

Worrying about what can go wrong is understandable, especially for parents of newborns. But what may go wrong is not very different from what happens in ordinary living. For example, when your son falls off his bike, scrapes his knee at the playground, or cuts himself while slicing vegetables for dinner, he is at risk for bleeding, bruising, and infection. Circumcision carries the same risks.

When the foreskin is separated from the glans, and again, when the foreskin is cut off, there is risk of bleeding and a risk of infection—the same risks as when a boy scrapes his knee. In other words, not much serious risk. While the cut for a circumcision sounds scary, it rarely causes more than minor bleeding (which can be treated by applying pressure) or a minor infection (which can be treated with an antibiotic cream). This low-risk level is especially true when the circumcision is performed on a healthy infant, by a trained, licensed, experienced circumciser who pays a great deal of attention to hygiene.

The American Academy of Pediatrics (AAP) estimates that only 2 percent of routine neonatal circumcisions involve post-procedure bleeding or infection, and most instances are minor. The American Academy of Family Physicians (AAFP) estimates a complication rate ranging from 0.1 percent to 35 percent, most involving infection, bleeding, or failure to remove enough of the foreskin. A common consensus figure is that between 2 and 5 percent of circumcisions involve some kind of complication. One pediatrician, who has practiced for over forty years, told us he has never encountered a serious complication after circumcision, although he has seen a number of poorly done circumcisions. So yes, you can expect your son's glans to look bloody after his foreskin has been cut off. You can also expect that he will recover quickly. Within days the wound will have healed, and within a week or so the glans will have healed and any bruising will have faded.

On the other hand

Occasionally, even a tiny cut or minor surgical procedure erupts into a major medical problem. For example, we've all read stories about raging infections from manicures, usually because an instrument had been inadequately sanitized. We know of a 14-year-old who had routine oral surgery to prepare for braces, hemorrhaged pints of blood and nearly lost her life. And, the American Academy of Family Physicians reported a mortality rate of 1 in a study of 500,000 circumcisions—a small percentage, but an enormous tragedy for that infant's family. So yes, there are horror stories for any surgical procedure, no matter how minor. And yes, we just broke our promise not to repeat any.

While horror stories about circumcisions are easy to find, especially on the Internet and in newspapers, we don't advise factoring them into circumcision decision-making. Why? Because they are rare. We can say, after much research, that most circumcisions are uneventful—especially when the circumcision is performed by a medically-trained, experienced circumciser. Afterward, you are most likely to go home with a healthy, circumcised infant, who has a piece of Vaseline-coated gauze on his penis, and who will heal rapidly.

A little more perspective

Medical procedures, like many activities in life, carry risks. Think about television ads for pharmaceutical products. After convincing viewers of the product's benefits, the ads list (because laws say they must) every risk of taking the product. It's a wonder that any antihistamine, acne medication or other product ever earns consumer confidence. The simple answer is: because the promised benefits appear to outweigh the risks.

The most common risks in infant circumcision are, again: bleeding, bruising, and infection. There are some more alarming risks—such as the possibility that the circumciser will accidentally cut into the glans. This can cause excessive bleeding and, in extreme events, partial amputation of the glans. This risk is greatly reduced if the circumciser uses a protective device, such as the Gomco clamp, or the Plastibell, which are designed to eliminate the risks of cutting into a glans. And, we repeat: the risks are reduced if you use a trained, experienced, certified circumciser or physician.

Treating a complication

Treatments for the most common complications that occur during or after circumcision are generally simple and effective.

Bleeding and bruising

Whenever the skin is cut, some bleeding and bruising may result. Circumcision is no exception, but bleeding and bruising are less likely if the foreskin has already (naturally) separated from the glans. The use of a circumcision clamp helps control bleeding since it stems the flow of blood to the foreskin. Minor bleeding can usually be stopped by applying pressure and bruises will gradually fade without treatment. Significant bleeding is rare, and may indicate a clotting disorder. This would require medical attention

After the foreskin has been removed, the glans is often wrapped in gauze to protect it from abrasion while healing. Unscented Vaseline can be applied to soothe and protect the glans.

Infection

Because the wound takes time to heal, an infection can sometimes occur. Usually, a minor infection can be treated with a topical antibiotic cream. Sometimes, but rarely, a more serious infection can develop—such as a staph (staphylococcal) infection. Just the names of these infections—for example: MRSA, which stands for Methicillin-resistant Staphylococcus aureus—are enough to alarm anyone. MRSA and some other serious staph infections can be resistant to antibiotics. Thus prevention—by excellent hygiene—is important during and after a circumcision and while the wound is healing.

Urinary tract infections (UTIs)

There is much debate over circumcision and UTIs and other infections. Some studies indicate a slightly lower risk of UTIs for circumcised infants (a recent American Academy of Pediatrics study showed that 1 percent of intact infants will develop a UTI in the first year, compared to .1 percent of circumcised infants). However this advantage may be counterbalanced by the risks of the circumcision procedure itself. Other studies show different statistics and many studies are criticized for not taking other factors into account, or for being biased or not adequately rigorous. Rather than overwhelm you with the results of many inconclusive or contradictory studies, we suggest you consult your physician and pediatrician.

Both circumcised and intact infants can develop a urinary tract infection, due to an abnormality of the tract or exposure to bacteria. Occasionally a UTI will occur while the circumcision is healing—perhaps because the parents are timid in washing around the healing penis, or a cut or abrasion on the penis or glans becomes infected, and the infection spreads into the urinary tract. Feces in the infant's diaper can cause a

UTI. Most UTIs are mild, and resolve themselves, or can be treated with an antibiotic.

Too little or too much foreskin cut off

This complication is sometimes subjective or aesthetic—much as the appraisal of a breast reduction can be. Did the surgeon take off too much, too little—or just enough?

Sometimes a parent—or fellow— will think that not enough of the foreskin was removed and that the penis doesn't look circumcised. If the boy was circumcised for a religious or cultural reason, he or his parents may wish to have more of the foreskin removed.

When too little foreskin tissue is cut away, leftover tissue can re-adhere to the glans or the penile shaft, and lead to the formation of skin bridges. This problem can be corrected with a minor follow-up procedure, or, if necessary, with a second circumcision.

Sometimes, when too little tissue is removed, the wound contracts and forms a ring of scar tissue. The ring may shrink back, and may then lead to phimosis—a tight foreskin—that will not allow the penis to achieve a comfortable erection, or sometimes makes urinating difficult. Surgery can correct this situation. Surgery can also remove any extra foreskin that gets stuck to a glans, or fix a frenulum that was not completely removed and which leaves the glans at an angle that makes urinating awkward.

A cutting "too-much" problem may occur if the circumciser removes the foreskin along with skin from the penile shaft. Part of the penile shaft may then be exposed and vulnerable to infection. Usually the situation corrects itself, as new skin grows and covers the wound. Occasionally the condition requires a skin graft.

Another problem may arise if too much foreskin or penile skin is removed. The male, as an adult, may find erections are painful, or appear distorted. A different problem may occur if the surgical scar from the circumcision is badly placed—although this is generally an aesthetic problem, not a medical issue.

Finally, and rarely, a condition called "concealed penis" may develop. This happens when the circumciser removes too much of the outer foreskin while leaving too much of the inner lining. The circumcision wound heals, but the inner layer continues to grow. This causes the penis to be pushed back, into the fat pad of the pubic area. The penis may then be concealed in the fat pad. In time the condition may resolve itself. If it doesn't, a surgery using a skin graft is performed, to allow the penis to protrude.

A rare situation

A few extremely traditional religious circumcisers continue to use ancient techniques that carry the risk of transmitting a serious infection—such as syphilis, TB, herpes or HIV/AIDs—to the infant during the circumcision. Specifically, after the foreskin is cut off, the circumciser uses his mouth to suck the blood away from the wound. Today, most traditional circumcisers sponge off the blood. Still, we occasionally read of this dangerous practice being used and resulting in disease transmission and the death of the infant. Indeed, these are the stories that make headlines and they are also the stories that lead public health officials to implore traditional circumcisers to use only medically safe, hygienic circumcision techniques. Use a physician or licensed, certified circumciser and avoid this risk.

Precautions

Significant bleeding is rare, as we mentioned earlier. It may be a sign of a clotting disorder. If a parent or close family relative has a clotting disorder, the infant can be tested before the procedure and precautions can be taken. If a baby has significant bleeding, treatment will be more quickly available if the procedure is in a hospital or medical facility.

So, again, we advise using an experienced doctor or a certified circumciser, who follows modern, sound medical practices. You may also want to check the safety and hygiene record of the hospital, medical facility or birthing center. And if you are planning to have the circumcision in your home or another non-medical setting, try to ensure that the setting is as sterile as possible.

Medical problems after circumcision

Once the foreskin and frenulum are removed, the skin on the glans toughens up a bit, making it less vulnerable to the small abrasions and irritations that may affect a more sensitive glans—especially during rough, dry sex. A tougher, circumcised glans is less likely to be irritated by sand, dirt, or coarse clothing. But if the circumcision was improperly performed, the glans may be tilted at an angle that makes urinating in a straight line or arc difficult. While this can be surgically corrected, the fellow who suffers from it is likely to find it bothersome, embarrassing, and a reason to wish that he had not been circumcised.

From statistics to real life

Now that you've read about the risks, we will throw a few statistics at you. As you read them, consider that they are based on all circumcisions, including those performed by inadequately trained circumcisers and by circumcisers in a hurry or working under stress. A young doctor, for example, told us that she once—at a respected medical center—faced a line-up of newborns waiting to be circumcised. Many were crying, especially those strapped tightly onto circumcision boards. While we trust, and our research suggests, that this situation is uncommon, it is conceivable that an inexperienced doctor or other circumciser, under this type of pressure, could make a mistake and cut off too much skin, or accidentally cut too far.

Every source we consulted offered a slightly different set of statistics about mishaps or complications. Not surprisingly, the choice of statistics often told us something about the pro-circ, anti-circ, or un-biased stance of the source. For example, one source gives a complication rate of .02 per 1,000 circumcisions. In contrast, the American Academy of Family Physicians estimated the risk at 2 deaths per 1 million circumcisions. One widely accepted statistic is that the risk of any complication is 0.2 to 2 percent in all circumcisions. These complications include minor bleeding, infection, and more serious events such as damage to the glans and even death. But when you look at the figures in each study (and perhaps jump to a conclusion), consider whether the study was tabulating deaths or total risks.

Before you decide not to circumcise because of the 1 death per 500,000 circumcisions, consider that this statistic included all circumcisions—on infants, boys, and men. While the infants' circumcisions were probably elective, the others may have been to correct problems.

Another consideration is that statistics of circumcision risks generally do not take into account the risk of remaining intact, such as the risk of a kidney infection, which is greater in intact than in circumcised infants (although it is still a small risk).

By now, it should be obvious that it is easy to get confused by statistics. This is often because the various sources measure risks and report statistics differently. A safe conclusion seems to be that if a circumcision is performed properly—by a trained, licensed, experienced circumciser, who follows all hygiene, health, and safety precautions—it is a relatively safe procedure that leads to few, mostly minor, complications, most of which are easily remedied. Again, the risks depend on the technique and equipment used, the hygiene standards, the circumciser's skill, depth of experience and training, and even his or her stamina on the circumcision day. The risks also depend on the quality of aftercare.

Cautions, again

As we mentioned earlier, if someone in either parent's family—parent, grandparent, aunt, or uncle, or sibling—has a bleeding disorder or a history of heavy bleeding after a minor procedure, or if either parent is adopted and has no information about his or her birth parents' medical history, you might want to delay circumcision until the infant can be tested for a bleeding problem. Or you can forego or postpone circumcision.

If your son has a malformation of the penis, he should not be circumcised since his foreskin tissue may be needed to correct it. Circumcision for a premature or below-normal birthweight infant should be delayed until the infant is considered sturdy enough. With a thorough exam to determine an infant's health and enough time to judge his stability (a reason some suggest delaying a circumcision to the biblically prescribed eighth day after birth), and with knowledge of the family's medical history, you can reduce the risks of circumcision a great deal. Finally, as a last precaution, if you can't find a skilled, experienced circumciser, postpone the circumcision until you find one.

Worry now or worry later

That "life is a gamble" is too trite a statement to insert into this debate. It might help, however, to consider what kind of gambler you are. If you're totally risk-avoidant, you can decide to avoid the risks of circumcision. But then you will assume the risks of leaving the child intact. Clearly, neither choice is risk-free. Fortunately, neither decision incurs a great risk—a point to remember when you are weighing the statistics on both sides of the issue.

To wrap up

In the big picture, circumcision is a minor surgical procedure, with rather low risks. As medical procedures go, circumcisions are easy to learn, easy to master, and rarely have complications. So, while 1 in 300 to 500 infants may have a minor problem—slight bleeding or a minor infection—299 to 499 infants will have no problems. Remember that these figures include procedures by circumcisers with far less experience than your circumciser will (should!) have. They may include procedures for boys and men with conditions that required a circumcision to cure a problem, not prevent one.

Yes, we are optimistic, and we believe statistics indicate that your son is unlikely to face significant complications during or after a circumcision.

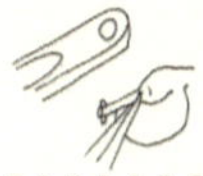

SECTION TWO

Religious, cultural & personal issues

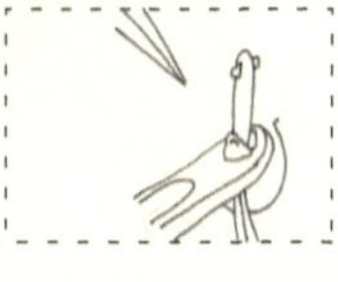

CHAPTER FIVE

Circumcising for religion

Honoring a religious or cultural tradition is perhaps the oldest and most often mentioned reason for deciding to circumcise—especially among Jews and Muslims. For some parents, circumcision is a personal religious choice.

For others, it may be important to the spouse or partner, or to the infant's grandparents. This is a big topic, and we discuss it more fully on our website: theCircumcisionDecision.com. Here, we will focus on the basic religious issue, which is: What is your responsibility to your son and how essential is circumcision to his religious tradition?

In Jewish tradition

> This is my requirement that you and your descendants after you must keep: Every male among you must be circumcised. You must circumcise the flesh of your foreskins. This will be a reminder of the covenant between me and you. Throughout your generations every male among you who is eight days old must be circumcised, whether born in your house or bought with money....The sign of my covenant will be visible in your flesh as a permanent reminder. Any uncircumcised male who has not been circumcised in the flesh of his foreskin will be cut off from his people—he has failed to carry out my requirement.
>
> – Genesis, 17:10-14

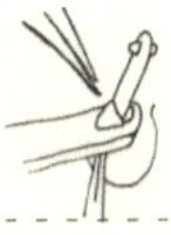

This sounds like a pretty clear directive until you consider that in the Book of Exodus, Moses—the patriarch of all patriarchs, the towering figure in the Torah—fails to circumcise his two sons, who were born to Zipporah, his beautiful, non-Jewish wife. If it was okay for Moses not to circumcise his sons, is it okay for you? Ah, if you are Jewish or are married to or partnered with someone Jewish, you probably know that question can yield a variety of conflicting, yet logical responses.

In the beginning of Judaism

Abraham is said to have circumcised himself, his servants, his son Ishmael and his son Isaac. And he made a pact with God that he, and all the Jews who followed him, would circumcise their sons or find someone to circumcise them. This was the deal Abraham literally cut with God, for in those days, deals were sealed by a cut. An animal was slaughtered and split in half. Both parties to the deal passed between the two halves of the animal, sealing the deal in blood. Thus, the Covenant of Abraham is the sealing of the deal. God promised to bless Abraham and his descendants and give them land, and Abraham promised that he and his people would obey God's commandments and mark the foreskins of future generations as a sign of that covenant.

Thus, according to Jewish law, every Jewish father is required to circumcise his sons. If he cannot fulfill that duty, his wife is expected to, and if she can't, his son (later) or his community is to assume the responsibility. From ancient Judaism, and through thousands of years of

Jewish history, circumcision remains a parental *duty*, not a choice. For modern Jews, including Reform and secular Jews, it is a choice.

However, it is a choice that is expected to be informed, thoughtful, carefully considered, and mindful of Jewish law and tradition. No Jew is ever expected to circumcise an unhealthy infant.

Now here's the "small print." To fulfill the religious obligations of Jewish circumcision, there are certain requirements. First, the circumcision is to be performed during daylight, on the eighth day of the infant's life. This timing is so important that it can take place on the Sabbath or on a Jewish holiday, even Yom Kippur. Second, the circumcision should not be just a medical procedure, but should be part of a religious ceremony, called a Bris, or Brit Milah, that includes traditional Jewish blessings and a Hebrew naming. The circumciser could be a mohel, a trained Jewish circumciser who can recite the Hebrew blessings. Or, a rabbi or cantor or other Jewish participant can say the blessings and do the naming while a doctor or other qualified person performs the circumcision.

For Jews observing Jewish law strictly, especially Orthodox and many Conservative Jews, there are other requirements. The foreskin should be removed with one circular cut, and some blood must be shed—because circumcision is fulfillment of a covenant, which requires the seal of blood.

If you are reluctant to have your infant son circumcised in front of family members and friends, you can choose to have him circumcised in a hospital, or birthing center, or a doctor's office, or at home, or elsewhere, without the bris and not necessarily on the eighth day. Note that this will fulfill the Jewish cultural tradition but will not fulfill the religious requirements. To fulfill those, you can have a private circumcision, with someone to recite the prayers and do the Hebrew naming. (Circumcision does not require the presence of a minyan of ten adults.) Or, you can have the circumcision privately, and then have a token amount of blood taken at the bris.

In a response to an unsuccessful 2011 attempt to ban neonatal circumcision in San Francisco, the major Reform Jewish organization—the Union of Reform Jews (URJ)—issued a resolution reaffirming the ritual of circumcision. They decried the proposed ban as an attack on religious freedom. Thus, while Reform Judaism accepts driving and working on the Sabbath, eating non-Kosher foods and marriage to a non-Jew, it insists on maintaining the oldest tradition in Judaism—circumcision.

Now, you may ask, what happens to the son of a Jewish father who chooses not to circumcise the boy? If his mother is Jewish, the son will be considered Jewish by Orthodox and other traditional Jews. Orthodox Jews will, however, expect the son to get himself ritually circumcised, meaning, at a *bris*, when he is an adult. In contrast, Reform Jews believe that even with a foreskin, if the child has one Jewish parent—mother or father—he can be Jewish. But, *only* if he is raised Jewish and makes a public commitment to Judaism. The public commitment means he will need some Jewish education, a Bar Mitzvah or Confir mation, and other public acts of Judaism, such as a trip to Israel and observance of Jewish holidays.

And, according to URJ's recent resolution, he will need to be circumcised someday. Reform Judaism, however, no longer requires converts to Judaism to be circumcised.

Perhaps one reason Jews maintain the tradition of circumcising newborns is because rabbis and scholars know that a Jew who isn't circumcised at birth is less likely to have himself circumcised later. This may be generally true, but we note that hundreds of thousands of Jewish males born behind the Iron Curtain after World War II were barred from being circumcised, but they later chose to be circumcised when they were allowed to emigrate to the U.S., Israel, Europe, and elsewhere during the 1970s and 80s.

Our advice

We suggest that if you decide to circumcise your son because he is Jewish, then fulfill the basic Jewish requirement to have the circumcision performed on the eighth day, by a doctor, a doctor/mohel, or by a certified circumciser. If the circumciser cannot recite the blessings and do the Hebrew naming, ask someone who can to fulfill this function. Our further advice may offend Orthodox Jewish rabbis. This is that we strongly advise using a physician/mohel or a physician, accompanied by a rabbi or cantor. Our reasons are: (1) a mohel who is not a physician is limited to topical pain relief, not injectable pain relief which is much more effective. Some mohels rely only on wine for pain relief, claiming (often and wrongly) that infants do not register pain. (2) A physician circumciser will use a circumcision shield, such as the Gomco shield, to protect the glans from being accidentally cut or severed. A mohel may use the Mogen shield, which doesn't offer total protection from an accidental cutting of the glans. And (3) because a few, very traditional Orthodox mohels still follow the practice of sucking the blood from the penis, which can put the infant at risk for a serious, even fatal, infection.

In the Muslim tradition

Unlike Jewish circumcision, which is prescribed by law in Judaism's holy book, the Torah, circumcision for Muslims is not mandated by Islam's holiest book, the Qur'an. The Muslim requirement is based on the Sunnah, Mohammad's recorded words and actions, and on the Hadith, the narrative of his life. In the Sunnah, it is written that Mohammad stated that circumcision is a "law for men…."

Most Muslims follow the tradition of Mohammed, who is said to have been born without a foreskin, and who is also said to have issued five rules of hygiene. The first is that males should be circumcised. The rest relate to mature males: they should shave their pubic hair, trim their mustaches, cut their fingernails and pluck their armpit hairs. Clearly, to Muslims, personal cleanliness is essential for holiness and is a primary reason for circumcision. Also, many Muslims desire to follow the example, or the path, of Mohammad in all things. For most Muslims, circumcision is considered an introduction to the Islamic faith and is a sign of being a member of the Islamic community. Today the majority of Muslim males are circumcised

Unlike Jews, Muslims do not have a universal, established ritual for circumcision or a universal tradition for when, where and how a male is circumcised. Nor is there a fixed age, although most Muslim boys are circumcised some time before puberty. The age varies by country, region, sect and even family. Today many Muslims, especially those living within Western cultures, have their sons circumcised in a hospital, by a physician, on the seventh day of the infant's life. Others have their sons circumcised during childhood, perhaps when they start religious school or when they have learned to recite the entire Qur'an. Still others have their sons circumcised before puberty or prior to marriage. One reason for circumcising boys at an older age is so that they will remember their circumcision and also, perhaps, because their wish to appear strong before their friends will help them through the ordeal. The boy's father, grandfather, uncles and others support him and offer comfort, and then congratulate him on his bravery.

In some countries, Muslims celebrate a circumcision with a lavish party, attended by family and friends, who bring gifts for the boy. Sometimes a boy is circumcised along with other boys who are relatives or friends. In rural settings, Muslims may have their sons circumcised quietly, by the town circumciser.

For parents making an interfaith or cross-cultural circumcision decision, or for Muslim parents considering not circumcising, a Muslim cleric or someone in the family group may be able to offer advice.

While the decision might seem hard, these parents do have the advantage of time since, in the Muslim tradition, there is no requirement to circumcise boys as infants.

In the Christian tradition

Learning when and why Christians abandoned circumcision was one of the most interesting areas of research for us. Condensing (or omitting) centuries of history, we'll get to the point: Christians abandoned the Covenant of Abraham, the law for circumcision, because they did not think circumcision necessary for spiritual purity. They believed that "circumcising the heart"— removing the impurities and blemishes that tarnish the soul—was the pathway to spiritual purity and to being connected to Christ, the Messiah. This circumcision of the heart is achieved by baptism and immersion in water—not by cutting of a foreskin.

Jesus, born Jewish, was circumcised on the eighth day after birth. After his death, his disciples convened, around 50 CE, to discuss the future of Christianity. They decided to heed the Apostle Paul's advice to abandon infant circumcision. Paul also advised doing away with the requirement for converts to be circumcised. In fact, Paul convinced his followers to separate from Judaism. Instead of converting to Christian Judaism, they would become Christians, who shared roots with Jews but no longer shared their laws or traditions—including the tradition of circumcision and laws governing food.

In time, Christians came to abhor circumcision, and eventually condemned and outlawed it. Jews could circumcise sons, but were prohibited from circumcising converts. If they were found guilty of circumcising a convert, they could be tortured or put to death, along with their entire community. In Spain, during the fourteenth and fifteenth centuries, Jews were forced to convert to Christianity, or were expelled and banned from circumcising their sons. Some brave conversos (the name given to Jews who converted to Christianity) secretly circumcised their infant sons.

Ironically, the development of germ theory and an understanding of the importance of hygiene later led many Christians, especially in the United States and the British Commonwealth, to adopt circumcision. However, these Christians did not embrace the religious tradition of circumcision.

In the U.S., circumcision remains popular in the general population; although the rates have fallen for various reasons, including the fact that many medical plans—especially state-funded plans—won't pay for routine circumcisions. In Europe, most non-Jews and non-Muslims leave their infants intact. So, if you are a Christian married to a Jew or a Muslim, the religious issue will not affect you. But it may be an issue for your partner or spouse or your in-laws. Thus, learning more about why circumcision is an important religious tradition may help you to help them grapple with it.

Other religions and cultures

A few other religions and cultures circumcise male children as a rite of passage into manhood. The custom of circumcision is widespread through African nations and among Australian Aborigines, Coptic Christians, Ethiopian Orthodox Christians, the Druze, Pacific Islanders, and others. Latinos and Asians generally leave males intact.

In ancient cultures in Africa and Australia, males living in hot, desert conditions may have embraced circumcision for reasons similar to those of the Egyptians, Babylonians, Jews and others: hygiene, fertility and aesthetics, and to promote clan identification and solidarity, and perhaps as a remnant of sacrificial and religious rituals.

Around the world, and in your life, too

It is estimated that 20 to 35 percent of all males, worldwide, are circumcised, primarily for religious and cultural reasons, although religion and culture are often intertwined. Religious elements are transformed into cultural practices—and vice versa.

For example, many Jews who don't go to temple, light Sabbath candles or keep kosher homes circumcise their sons for the sake of tradition—Jewish tradition, that is. Muslims willing to adopt modernity still circumcise sons, although increasingly not as rite of passage, but as infants, in a physician's office.

Although Jews and Muslims constitute only 3 to 5 percent of the U.S. population, 60 to 80 percent of U.S. males are circumcised. This means that many Christians, Buddhists, Mormons, atheists, agnostics and others are circumcising for non-religious reasons (although some may be circumcising because a son's other parent wants the child circumcised for a religious reason).

For a variety of reasons—such as costs, or the desire to follow a natural life style—many U.S. parents (especially those on the West Coast) are choosing not to circumcise newborns. However, among Jews and Muslims, circumcision remains the majority decision. Choosing to go against religious tradition may require defending your decision to your partner, your parents, your in-laws, and someday to your son, as well. Still, while you may be among the minority in your religion, you will certainly not be the first to question the religious tradition of circumcision.

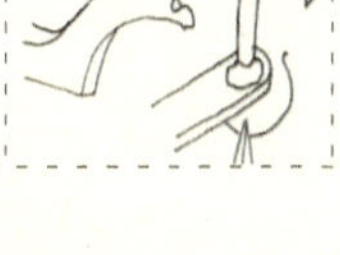

CHAPTER SIX

Circumcising for cultural reasons

As noted, 20 to 35 percent of males on this planet are circumcised, which means the majority of males are intact. Today, however, in the United States, Israel, Turkey, the Middle East, South Korea and many African nations, the majority of parents choose to circumcise their sons. While some make this choice for religious reasons, others just follow the custom in their community or culture.

In England, Scandinavia, Western Europe, Latin America, Asia and some other areas, most parents leave their infants intact—again, because that is what they see other parents do. Indeed, we found that most parents don't struggle with the decision. They do what is customarily done in their culture or religious tradition. Why buck tradition? Why challenge the norm?

Jews, even those who are not observant, often have their sons circumcised out of respect for tradition and their cultural ties to Judaism. They may skip the ritual ceremony but not the procedure. There are exceptions to this generalization—most commonly, Jews who question tradition, or who are in an interfaith or intercultural marriage.

Parents raised in a different culture, with different ideas about circumcision, approach the decision from their own cultural perspective. And since this book is for parents who want to make a rational, informed and conscious decision—one that may go against tradition

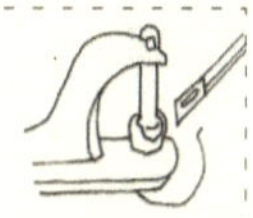

or a cultural norm—this chapter will look at circumcision through the lens of tradition and culture.

What is a cultural norm and why does it matter?

A cultural norm is defined as a commonly accepted pattern of behavior within a group, subgroup or society. The term "norm" sounds significant, but a norm can be about food preferences, dress codes, music choices, or any aspect of culture—from beliefs, attitudes and expectations to current slang. Unlike a set of laws, norms are not absolute, but they can be powerful, and wide-ranging. They influence many aspects of a culture, including how people worship, what they eat and how they greet, and how they bury their dead.

Following a cultural norm is usually easy, while defying the norm can be more difficult. Minor transgressions against the norm may lead to disapproval or mockery; while transgressions regarded as forbidden or "taboo" can lead to serious consequences, even banishment or death.

Sometimes the law reflects a cultural norm, as in Western societies where the cultural norm (and the law) allows only one spouse at a time, although it is legal to divorce a spouse and marry someone else, and even repeat that pattern. In contrast, another culture (and its laws) may allow someone, usually a male, to have more than one spouse at a time, but may make it difficult or impossible to divorce.

Norms about the body

Altering the penis—by removing part or all of the foreskin—is one of the earliest recorded forms of body-alteration. An Egyptian wall carving, dating from 2400 BCE, shows a priest cutting off a man's foreskin with a stone knife. In some ancient cultures in the Middle East and other regions, circumcision rituals were common, although their origins varied from one group to another. Some cultures circumcised for aesthetic reasons, believing that removing a foreskin enabled a male to "look perfect," and be pure and godlike. In other cultures, circumcision identified an elite class, such as when only circumcised and physically perfect males could be temple priests. Even in the United States, during the 1940s, circumcision served as a subtle class distinction, since many boys whose parents could afford hospital births were circumcised but boys born at home, in rural settings, were often left intact.

In a number of cultures, especially in Africa and Australia, circumcision served as a rite of passage into adulthood. In many cultures, it was—and is—a mark of kinship, of belonging to a clan, tribe or group. In still other cultures, it is a symbolic sacrificial act, or is considered necessary for achieving purity, or ensuring fertility. In contrast, many cultures, past and present, leave males intact and see the intact penis as aesthetically perfect.

When cultures rub against each other, perhaps because one culture conquers the other, or because of a massive migration, it is interesting to note which norms prevail. In Asia, for example, the norm was to leave men intact. When World War II ended in 1945, and the United

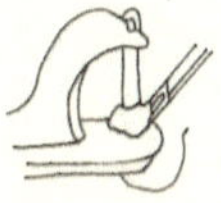

States Trusteeship of South Korea began, the U.S. cultural practice of circumcising spread through the society. Now, nine out of ten South Korean male high-school students are circumcised, usually during adolescence.

Many cultures that prefer to leave males intact will tolerate a subculture with a tradition of circumcising, and vice versa. Sadly, though, the convergence of cultures has sometimes resulted in tragedy. A conquering army has forcibly circumcised the defeated enemy. Or the victors have outlawed circumcision and imposed penalties on those who defied the ban.

A series of cultural twists

The United States has had an interesting cultural dance with circumcision. In 1791, just a few years after the formation of the nation, the Bill of Rights was ratified. It promoted a new cultural norm that guaranteed the free exercise of religion, and the separation of church and state. Although most of the young nation's citizens followed Christianity—a religion that had abandoned circumcision nearly eighteen centuries earlier—religious freedom created a tolerance for circumcision. However, in the primarily Christian society, the norm was to leave males intact.

Irony

Almost a century later, a great flood of immigrants, mainly from Europe, began arriving on U.S. shores. Among these tens of millions of immigrants were 2.5 million European Jews who arrived between 1881 and

1924. Many tried to assimilate, sometimes refusing to teach children their native language lest they sound like foreigners and be subject to taunting and discrimination.

For these Jews, the cultural norm, of course, was circumcision. In Europe, this religious tradition (among others—including clothing styles, food customs and Sabbath observance) had set the Jews apart, and at times subjected them to ridicule, disapproval or worse. In this new country, instead of being mocked or criticized, they found many Christians embracing circumcision—not for religious reasons but embracing it nonetheless. The same cultural shift was occurring in England, Ireland, and Australia, when Jewish immigrants arrived in those countries. It is ironic that many Christians, whose culture had condemned circumcision in earlier times, were now adopting the practice. What led to that change?

A key factor in this shift had origins in the field of medicine. By about 1870, a few prominent physicians in the U.S. and Western Europe became convinced that the foreskin caused a host of problems—especially childhood masturbation (termed "self-abuse" at the time). Masturbation was seen as a sinful act and, they believed, could cause insanity, blindness, epilepsy, tuberculosis, venereal disease and many other ailments. And, removal of the foreskin would prevent or cure these conditions, they claimed.

A number of medical discoveries seemed to support these ideas. Lewis Sayre, a surgeon and later a founder of the American Medical Society, gained attention in 1870 when he cured a paralyzed boy by a circumcision that freed the child's penis from a restricting foreskin (a condition now called phimosis). Louis Pasteur, a French chemist, discovered the role of bacilli in causing contagious infections; Robert Koch, a German surgeon and medical researcher, identified microscopic bacteria as the cause of specific diseases, including cholera and tuberculosis. The work of Sayre, Pasteur, Koch and others led to the formulation of the germ theory of disease—a theory that diseases and infections are often caused and spread from one person to another by microscopic bacteria.

With these discoveries, bodily emissions—including feces, blood and mucus—came to be seen as dirty and dangerous carriers of disease agents. Genitals, with sometimes foul-smelling smegma, were viewed as a medical menace. In fact, doctors made claims that eliminating the foreskin would protect the public from venereal disease, cancer, and many other miseries.

Previously, with little understanding of disease transmission, doctors and assistants were not trained to routinely scrub their hands before surgery. Thus, surgeons and obstetricians, in particular, could spread infections from one patient to another. With the teaching of germ theory, recognition of the importance of washing hands and personal hygiene—including penile hygiene, and the idea that a circumcised penis was cleaner—spread through the medical community and the general public.

In response to these discoveries, a public health system was organized, although it often lacked effective resources. This system zealously attacked disease with the few tools, techniques, and drugs available at the time, including quarantine (for tuberculosis), and folk medicine (including the use of cupping, leeches, potions and prayer), and surgery. Limited to these methods, doctors increasingly turned to circumcision as a weapon against infection.

In 1890, a comparative study of the health of American Jews was published in the *North American Review,* as "On the Vital Statistics of the Jews." This study provided an additional spur to the adoption of circumcision because it showed that the Jewish population (which circumcised all its males) had, on average, greater longevity, fewer stillborn children, a lower incidence of cancer and syphilis, and fewer "defective" children. Without any real cause-and-effect evidence, and little consideration of other factors such as social organization, sexual practices, ritual baths and routine hand-washing, neonatal circumcision gradually became the cultural norm in the U.S. and England.

Eventually, by the 1920s, a greater understanding of disease ended some of the baseless claims of circumcision's power. Still, the practice was promoted for good penile hygiene and prevention of conditions that do affect the penis, such as balanitis and phimosis.

One last, and interesting, factor that contributed to the acceptance of circumcision in the U.S. derived from the doctrines of some Protestant denominations that valued the Jewish roots of Christianity. These groups studied and came to respect the Old Testament, including its Covenant of Circumcision. Indeed, these Protestants, whose families had emigrated to the U.S. seeking religious freedom, respected the Jewish origins of Jesus and the tradition of his circumcision on the eighth day of his life. With that respect, came tolerance of the Jewish practice of circumcision.

Influenced by the promise of health benefits, both real and illusory; protected by the religious freedom guaranteed by the Bill of Rights (and still protected by that freedom); circumcision eventually—and ironically—became the cultural norm in the U.S. By 1950, nearly three out of four males were circumcised; by 1990, nearly nine out of ten were. Even immigrants from countries where the cultural norm had been to leave males intact had their infants and sometimes themselves circumcised—partly to assimilate and partly because they, too, wanted the health benefits many of their doctors believed would be gained.

Nothing stays the same

An August 17, 2010 headline in the *New York Times* read: "A Steep Drop Seen in Circumcision in the U.S.A." A federal health researcher reported that fewer than half the boys born in conventional hospitals from 2006 to 2009 were circumcised, in contrast to the two-thirds figure reported twenty years earlier. (These figures do not include boys circumcised in ritual circumcisions after leaving the hospital.)

Several factors account for that decrease. In our contemporary culture, rebellion itself has become a cultural norm. Our culture encourages change, diversity and tolerance. Some changes are reflected in popular culture, as tortillas, bagels and veggie burgers are now mainstream foods. Other changes have affected relationships and behavior. Cohabitation and having babies out of wedlock are common practices today. Young people have created new aesthetic norms, from tattoos, scarification and piercings to neon-colored hair and pubic-hair removal.

More and more people are finding reasons—and the courage—to challenge religious traditions and cultural norms, including the U.S. norm of circumcising male infants. Curiously, some new norms are a return to old ones—such as natural childbirth, midwife-assisted childbirth, breast-feeding, the family bed, and leaving the male penis intact. Some Jews, often those who choose organic, vegetarian or vegan food, value the environment and live "holistic" lives, are choosing to leave their sons intact—despite a tradition that has embraced circumcision for thousands of years.

With growing acceptance of cultural differences, and laws that support minorities and diversity, as well as the protections that have been earned by various rights movements—including women's rights, civil rights, gay rights, deaf rights and disabled rights, to name some—today's immigrants and foreign residents, who in the past might have adopted the U.S. norm to circumcise, are choosing to leave their sons intact.

Change in the medical community

Male circumcision is a common procedure, generally performed during the newborn period in the United States. In 2007, the American Academy of Pediatrics (AAP) formed a multidisciplinary task force of AAP members and other stakeholders to evaluate the recent evidence on male circumcision and update the Academy's 1999 recommendations

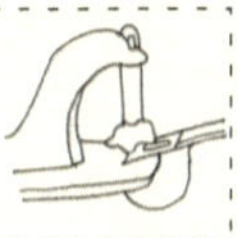

in this area. In late August, 2012, the AAP published an updated policy statement, which reflected a change from its earlier, neutral position on circumcision. The new statement supported the practice, stating that the evaluation of current evidence indicates the health benefits of newborn male circumcision outweigh the risks and that the procedure's benefits justify access to this procedure for families who choose it. Specific benefits identified included prevention of urinary tract infections, penile cancer, and transmission of some sexually transmitted infections, including HIV. The American College of Obstetricians and Gynecologists endorsed this statement.

Until this new policy statement, no major American or other national or international medical organization recommended neonatal circumcision. Opponents of infant circumcision are voicing objections and the impact of this revised policy statement remains to be seen.

A New Movement

Since the 1980s, a few doctors and psychologists have joined movements to oppose routine circumcision, and a few pediatricians, obstetricians and midwives now refuse to perform routine circumcisions. Some have created organizations and websites to inform the public about the full range of circumcision issues, including the benefits-versus-risks question, the importance of preventing pain and trauma, the choice of hospital versus ritual home procedures, the choice of circumciser and infants' rights. Some offer support to adults who lament their own circumcisions. And some support the recent activism to ban routine circumcision, although to date, these attempts have failed.

Money as an issue

In 1949, in Great Britain, where routine infant circumcision was nearly as popular as in the U.S., the British National Health Service stopped paying for hospital circumcisions. This policy change probably contributed to the decreased circumcision rate and today, less than one percent of British newborns are circumcised in the hospital in a culture that had embraced circumcision as a cultural norm a few decades earlier.

In the U.S., no doubt due in part to medical organizations' non-supportive position on routine infant circumcisions, about twenty states, including all the Western states, no longer allow state Medicaid funding for routine hospital circumcisions. A few private insurance companies have also stopped paying for newborn circumcisions, and most refuse to pay for elective (non-medical) circumcisions for older children and adults. The new AAP policy statement may lead to changes in some coverage.

Each of these factors—lack of medical endorsement, a return to seeing the intact penis as perfect, less pressure to assimilate and lack of funding for circumcisions—has contributed to a decrease in circumcision rates, especially on the West Coast, which has significant Latino and Asian-American populations and where fewer than 40 percent of male infants are being circumcised. Yet in other areas, especially the Midwest and the South, circumcision has remained common, with about eight out of ten male infants being circumcised. Overall, circumcision remains the the norm in the U.S, although the percentage of male infants being circumcised has been dropping.

Perhaps, if the cultural norm to circumcise becomes as dominant as it once was, the states and private insurance companies would feel pressure to pay for circumcisions. But perhaps not.

Enough about other people—what about you and your son?

The question to ask is: How important are cultural norms to you and your partner? You cannot predict whether or how much our cultural norms will change, or in which direction. You cannot predict what your son will be like as an adolescent or adult—where he will live, what he will do, who he will choose as partner. Actually, it is difficult to predict *anything* for our fast-moving, fast-changing society. All we can know is what the cultural norm is here and now.

You may be reading this book because you are considering challenging your society's or your family's norm. Or, you may be wrestling with the circumcision issue because you and your partner are from different cultures, with different cultural norms about circumcision.

Clearly, a decision that conforms to a cultural norm is easier to make than one that goes against it. But recognizing the increasing diversity and tolerance for that diversity in our culture, as well as the rapidly changing aesthetic, sexual, and even family norms (with so many babies being conceived or born through surrogates or with sperm and egg donors, to same-sex partners and single parents or through adoptions) and our exposure to many different beliefs, values and ideas—going against a cultural norm today will probably cause few ripples. You may be called upon to defend your decision to parents or friends, but with social networking, it is easy to find support for defying a social norm, or for following one. And this will be true even if you choose to leave your son intact while living in a religious community that has a tradition of circumcision.

Circumcision has been practiced since antiquity and remains the norm for hundreds of millions of males, so choosing to circumcise your son to follow the cultural norm is unlikely to cause you—or him—anguish or sleepless nights. (We can't be absolutely certain about this.) Leaving your son intact places him among the majority of males in the world, so even if that decision differs from your cultural norm, it should also not cause sleepless nights. First, he can choose to be circumcised later. Secondly, with many people now straying from cultural norms, and the increasing diversity of our society, it is less and less likely that your son will be the only intact male in his circle of friends or in the locker room. And, to repeat, he can reverse that decision on his own.

There are other reasons for choosing to circumcise or leave your son intact, aside from cultural norms—as we discuss through this book. Basing the decision on a wish to conform to culture, especially when it involves a private body part, carries less weight than it did twenty or fifty years ago. An intact son may be in a minority, but it will be a significant minority. Even if he eventually lives in a country where only

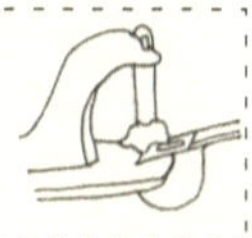

two percent of males are circumcised, as in some countries in Western Europe and Asia, minority groups (especially Jews and Muslims) within those countries have been defying that norm for centuries. While their sons may be considered "different," their penises are not likely to be the focus of the distinction. More likely it will be the cultural habits that they display on their sleeves and faces and in their daily lives, rather than those they tuck into their underwear.

U.S. Circumcision Rates

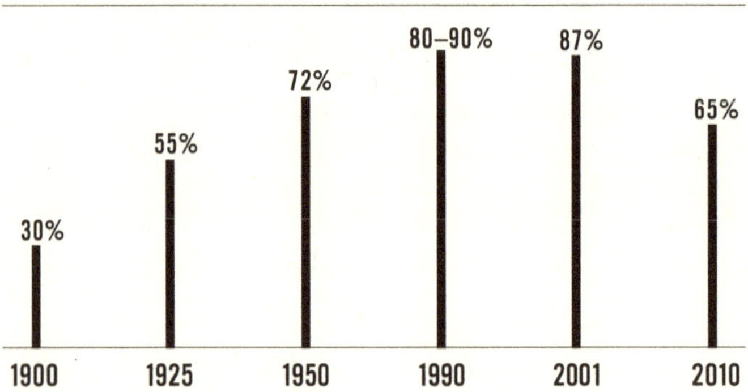

CHAPTER SEVEN

Is it important to look like Dad?

"So he will look like his father" is one of the most common reasons we hear people give for a decision to circumcise or not circumcise a son. "I want him to look like me," say many fathers. "I want him to look like his dad," say many mothers.

And sometimes:

I want him to look like his brother.

I want him to look like the other boys.

I want him to look like the men in his family.

To those who don't wrestle with the circumcision decision, the question of whether their son's penis should look like his father's might not seem important. It's a "non-issue," as the current phrase explains. But for others, it can be the key issue, the factor that determines the fate of their son's foreskin.

Here is an example. Janice is Jewish. Her husband is Lutheran. He was Lutheran—and intact—when they dated, and when they married. One recent day, Janet joined a few friends for lunch. Because of one friend's new baby, the conversation turned to circumcision and the question of "looking like Dad." Janice volunteered that her husband, Paul, wasn't circumcised, nor were her sons. They looked like

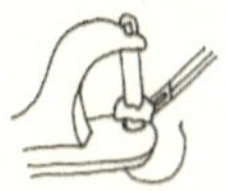

their father. One woman reported what her sons had told her—that in locker rooms and bathrooms, boys and men don't look around at other males. Those who do look risk being thought of as a pervert, or as someone "looking for action." So, in a public bathroom or locker room, whether your son's penis looks like everyone else's penis is unlikely to be a big issue—unless he is in middle school, when he might feel self-conscious no matter how he looks. But as Stephan, who grew up in a small town in the Midwest, with an intact penis (because his mother wanted him to look like his European father), told us, "What kid doesn't feel self-conscious about something? Part of growing up is learning how to be comfortable with who you are and how you look."

Why your son doesn't have to look like his father

Joshua is adopted and looks nothing like his father, brother, uncles or cousins. He is taller and thinner, and has straight hair in contrast to their curls. Perhaps you are expecting us to compare his penis to theirs. Well, we won't. When Joshua was asked if his penis looks like this dad's, he said: " I don't know."

Four-year-old Charlie is intact, while his father is circumcised. Until he was three, Charlie slept in his parents' bed, and still occasionally climbs into their bed. His family shares one bathroom, so Charlie often urinates while his dad shaves and his dad urinates when Charlie is bathing. Charlie isn't shy, and talks a lot. Never once has Charlie asked why his penis looks different from his father's.

Personal stories do not substitute for a scientific study. But anecdotal material can be informative. In several surveys where sexually active women were asked if their sexual partners were intact or circumcised, many women did not know. They had not thought about it much, and never noted a difference. One woman had to look at sketches of a penis with a foreskin and one without before she could answer the question. This is consistent with surveys reporting that some women prefer an intact penis, but many women don't know the difference and don't care. (As a historical note, an early study of whether circumcision prevented disease transmission was discredited after doctors discovered that many of the women in the study did not know whether or not their partners were circumcised.)

Our point is that what seems to be a big issue may not be so big. Fathers may care more about their sons looking like them, rather than the sons care about looking like their fathers. After all, a boy looks so different from an adult man (larger genitals, chest and pubic hair, muscles and all the other signs of maturity), would the difference in penises even register?

While circumcision may be an issue for your son someday, we don't think it is as significant as the issue many adopted children face: that of looking different from their adoptive parents, especially if they are of a different race or ethnicity. What makes people feel comfortable about their differences is being loved and accepted for who they are.

Foreskin or no foreskin doesn't seem a big deal in the whole picture of what and who you are. If a Jewish or a Muslim boy has a health

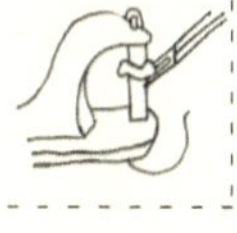

problem that precludes circumcision, his penis will not look like the others in his family. But he could still look like a family member. His penis won't show in family photographs, at the dinner table, at a class reunion, or in any public place.

Suppose you think you should circumcise your son because the majority of males in your town or your region are circumcised, and you don't want him to be the only intact boy in school. With declining circumcision rates and greater diversity in school populations, he may be in the minority but he is unlikely to be the only intact boy. He could, conceivably, be the only intact boy at a Jewish camp or school. As an adult, if he feels uncomfortable, or becomes part of an Orthodox community, he can choose to be circumcised then.

After consideration, we don't think that having a limp penis (erect they all look pretty much alike) that looks different from a dad's should be important—unless you expect your son to be a porn star, hang out at nudist colonies or attend San Francisco's Folsom Street Fair. So, no, we don't think concern about looking different should carry much weight. If you leave a son intact, and he is the only intact boy at Camp Wise or on a temple's Birthright trip to Israel, suggest a comeback if anyone teases him, such as: "Dude, let's get it straight… you are laughing at *me* because *you* got a part of your penis cut off?"

As for gym class, many schools have dispensed with after-gym-class showers, and many schools have replaced open showers with private stalls. Also, after middle school or high school, foreskins are rarely a topic of concern. The size of the penis, maybe. The presence or absence of a foreskin, probably not. In interviews with a number of intact young men who grew up in communities where most boys were circumcised, few reported teasing from locker-room buddies, classmates, girlfriends, or anyone else. We think the reverse is true, too. Intact males don't tease circumcised friends. Today it's OK to be different—or at least to have a penis that looks different. We hope other differences won't matter much ten or fifteen years from now, either.

The ugly past

Yes, looking circumcised—and therefore looking Jewish—during the Nazi period in Europe, sealed the fate of millions of Jewish males. "Never again" is what Jews and others say of the Holocaust. But a circumcised penis is unlikely to again seal a male's fate—at least not in the U.S., because circumcision is no longer a distinguishing characteristic. Many men, of different backgrounds, are circumcised (although circumcision rates are falling). Today a simple swab test reveals more about a person's genetic heritage than does a foreskin. The fact that Jewish men's circumcisions led to their deaths during the Holocaust and in previous eras of persecution is a reminder of a heinous crime—against Jews and against humanity.

The unknown

One reason you may want your son to look like his dad is because you admire his father. You want him to admire his father, also, and you think he may want to look like him. But what will having a penis like his father's penis do? Will the bond between them be strengthened? We hate to play with a cliché, but it is apt—the bond between a father and son is more than foreskin-deep. The bond grows from love and respect, from how a father treats a son when pleased or displeased, what a father and son do together, learn together, share. The quality of their relationship is based on factors stronger than the presence or absence of a foreskin. We doubt that a son will feel inferior if he is intact and his father is not. If he does, when he grows up, he can get circumcised to look like his dad.

Finally we believe that the decision to circumcise or leave a son's penis intact—for medical or health reasons, or religious or cultural reasons—is an important decision. Making the decision so that his penis will match his dad's is basing an important decision on a factor that doesn't really seem that important.

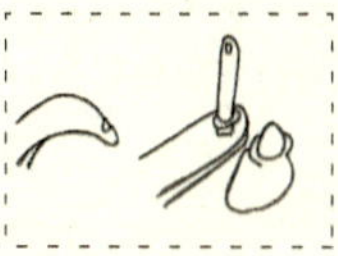

CHAPTER EIGHT

Is sex better with—or without—a foreskin?

The issue of sex with a foreskin versus sex without a foreskin is complicated and controversial. How does circumcision affect sex? Does it improve it? Damage it? Have no effect?

Oddly, a frequently cited reason—used both for leaving a foreskin intact and for removing it, and used both by men and by their partners—is the effect on sex. We've heard strong opinions from many on all sides of the question. We aim to discuss the issue frankly, but thinking about the future sexual behavior of an infant may be difficult.

Foreskins and sex

At the center of the debate over which is better—sex with a foreskin or sex without it—is the issue of sensitivity. Is sensitivity lost when a foreskin is removed? How much? Does that loss impact a man's sexual experience?

Foreskins, especially their inner linings and tips, are extremely sensitive to touch. Since we know that there are tens of thousands of nerve endings in both the outer and the inner foreskin, this is not surprising. Nor is it surprising that for many men (with or without a foreskin), a touch on the penis is enough to cause arousal. Sometimes just the thought or anticipation of being sexually aroused can cause an erection. The glans also has thousands of nerve endings, so a touch there can cause an erection, too. In summary, we can't provide a definitive answer to this part of the debate

Foreskins contribute to the sexual experience by their role in providing the natural lubricant called smegma. Circumcised males may produce less smegma. Is this a negative or a positive factor? Interestingly, those opposing circumcision regret the loss of smegma, while those favoring circumcision welcome the reduced smegma production! Why these opposite reactions? Some people prefer circumcised men as sexual partners because smegma can acquire a foul smell—especially if it is allowed to accumulate and grow stale. Some partners say smegma is a turn-off during oral sex. Yet other partners say they enjoy the natural lubrication that smegma provides, and that they are not turned off by it, even during oral sex. Given the wide variations among people and what turns some on and some off, these contradictory feelings are not really surprising.

A major reason foreskins may enhance the sexual experience is through their movement back and forth over the glans and penile shaft. This gliding movement provides pleasure for both the man and his partner. Some partners say that when the foreskin bunches up behind the glans corona, this adds to the pleasure of the sexual experience.

Many men, including circumcised men with loose circumcisions, use their extra skin to glide back and forth over their penis. Some men who are circumcised, as adults, and with a tight circumcision, state that losing that gliding motion isn't a big deal. Other men say that losing it is a big deal.

Some partners claim there is no comparison between sex with an intact man and sex with a circumcised man. (However, as we mentioned earlier, we have learned from a number of studies that many women don't know the circumcision status of a partner's penis.) Some partners have told us they think an intact man is hotter in bed, a lot hotter. But we want to remind you that a person's reason for dating or marrying one man over another or for choosing a life-partner, is rarely based on the presence or absence of a foreskin. And an intact man does have the option of being circumcised. The complex mixture of emotional components in a relationship, the love and caring, the sense of trust, are more important than opinion polls or survey results. Love seems to conquer all when it comes to foreskins or no foreskins.

Despite circumcised men's claims that they enjoy sex as much as intact men, and despite studies of men circumcised as adults, the question of whether a man enjoys sex more if intact or if circumcised, and whether a partner prefers an intact or a circumcised man, is impossible to answer. So forget about sex for a minute, and focus on a different appetite.

Some people have as few as 2,000 taste buds on the tongue. Others have 10,000. Do more taste buds make you a gourmet, capable of distinguishing the subtleties of fine cuisine? Or do extra taste buds make food taste too salty, too sweet or too anything? Responses to flavors and tastes depend on many details besides the number of taste receptors in your mouth—including the style of cooking you ate in your family home, your experiences tasting a range of cuisines, the atmosphere in a restaurant, the person sharing the meal with you, your mood before you tasted a morsel, and even the amount of time you spend eating, since rushing through a meal is no way to enhance the flavor of food. Like dining, sex is not just about filling a need, or about rushing as opposed to savoring. (Granted, though, at times rushing, like fast food, can be pleasurable.) Sex involves more than intercourse, too.

Since ancient times, people of many cultures have aspired to elevate and enhance sexual life, especially within an enduring relationship. The early Jews may have been trying to accomplish this. Yes, they circumcised the foreskin for religious reasons, to fulfill a covenant. Yes, they may have circumcised the foreskin in the belief that it would improve fertility, hygiene and health. Yes, in some cultures it may have been a relic of a sacrificial rite. But in the teachings of some religious sages and philosophers, circumcision was valued as a way to help a man control his lust. They believed that lust-control would be good for a long-term marriage and good for other aspects of a man's life, including allowing him time to concentrate on religious study. Moses Maimonides, a twelfth-century Jewish philosopher, rabbi and physician, saw a connection between circumcision and dialing down on lust. "Circumcision simply counteracts excessive lust," he wrote, "for there is no doubt that circumcision weakens the power of sexual excitement, and sometimes lessens the natural enjoyment." He also mentioned the possible special attraction of an intact male when he wrote: "It is hard for a woman with whom an uncircumcised man has had sexual intercourse, to separate from him. This is, as I believe, the best reason for the commandment concerning circumcision."

Why would controlling lust be good for a relationship? Today you might think the opposite, especially since some marriages last many decades.

Interestingly, a recent study by University of Chicago researchers showed that circumcised men had a higher incidence of STDs. The researchers also found that circumcised men were more likely to engage in sexually adventurous behavior, to experiment more with sex. Note: this is not necessarily because the men are circumcised. It could be that a higher percentage of young men now leave home for college and graduate work, travel more, marry later, and tend to live in urban centers such as New York City, Chicago, Los Angeles and San Francisco. Any or all of these factors may contribute to a man being more sexually savvy.

So maybe Maimonides was wrong about lust. Maybe he mistook lust for the ability to have an early and perhaps intense orgasm. But if circumcision delays orgasm, if both circumcised and intact men understand what truly turns on their partners—in early marriage and decades later—perhaps being circumcised or intact has less significance. Instead of dialing down lust, perhaps circumcision merely dials down sensitivity at the cellular level (because of fewer nerve endings). Thus, it may allow and even enhance the other components of a satisfying sexual experience—from kissing and caressing to what the brain imagines. After all, two people can dance together but learning how to be a fabulous dance team takes practice, and relies on the brain and the heart, as well as the body.

Summing up the possible effects of circumcision on sex

Masturbation

Sex experts say the loss of a foreskin can make masturbation more work. They claim that because circumcision removes the lining of the foreskin, less natural lubricant (smegma, again) is produced. Also, a tight circumcision may leave the skin on the erect penis too tight to easily move up and down to stimulate the penis. But an intact foreskin also can be too tight to retract or to move up and down.

The foreskin's up-and-down movement over the penis makes masturbation easier, but a hand can achieve the same result. If you are uncomfortable thinking about your son playing with himself, or masturbating, remember that a boy's self-investigation and playing with his penis helps to achieve the necessary separation between the glans and the foreskin.

Ejaculation

A male can ejaculate more quickly when he has a foreskin. Because the foreskin is so sensitive, men with foreskins tend to experience orgasms more quickly than men without foreskins. Today, many couples practice tantra sex or use medications to prolong orgasms, so what is so great about coming sooner? If it takes a man longer, his partner will have more time to prepare for an orgasm. And another orgasm.

Good sex

Sex is as much between the ears as it is between the thighs. Sexual satisfaction is supported by good communication, good foreplay, mutual respect, patience and love. If you want your son to experience sex in a positive way, he will need to learn to control his lust, to restrain himself at times and be a thoughtful, unselfish lover. This isn't necessarily achieved through circumcision nor guaranteed by an intact foreskin.

Who says it is so?

You cannot know how your son will feel about being circumcised or being intact when he is eighteen, twenty-five or sixty-five. Some studies have investigated circumcision's effect on sex, but most involved a small number of participants, or were self-reporting or anecdotal surveys, and therefore somewhat unreliable. Numerous studies and surveys and anecdotal evidence indicate that it is impossible to determine whether a man will be more sexually satisfied with or without a foreskin. Men who have been circumcised at birth will never know the difference, although some women we interviewed made interesting comparisons. Some preferred intact men—especially if their first experiences were with them. Others preferred circumcised men.

Men who were circumcised as adults also made comparisons—but in some cases the need for a circumcision (perhaps a tight foreskin or a foreskin vulnerable to tearing) might have contributed to a sexual problem. In many studies of sexual satisfaction before and after circumcision, the results are divided—so no firm conclusions can be drawn, despite the fervently argued claims you may find on some less-than balanced Internet sites. Usually, a simple majority (meaning less than 60 percent) reported being more satisfied with sex after being circumcised. Still, a significant percentage (about 40 percent) reported being less satisfied. And a number of men reported no difference. They had been happy with sex when intact and were happy with sex when circumcised.

Gay men seem to have stronger feelings about being circumcised versus being intact. Interestingly, the preferences seem to be affected by where the men live. Unscientific sources tell us that in Germany, where the majority of men are intact, gay men seem to prefer circumcised men. But in New York City, where many men are circumcised, some reports indicate gay men prefer intact men. Others say the opposite. Perhaps "being different" heightens the sexual experience for some.

A non-conclusion, of sorts

Clearly, neither statistical nor anecdotal data can provide a definitive answer about the sexual impact of circumcision. Your son's sexual life will depend on him, on his partners, and even on the customs that prevail when he is ready for sex.

In our culture and these times, we see sex as not just for procreation—it is also for pleasure. A range of sexual activities are considered acceptable—between consenting partners. We know that men who are circumcised report having satisfactory, good, and great sex. As do intact men. Today there are many ways to improve sex if the status of the foreskin seems to have an impact, or for other issues. There are pills, sex education classes, books, videos, and websites that teach people how to enjoy sex more and how to be better lovers. To return to your decision about your son's foreskin, you can choose to rely on religious, cultural, or family traditions, or the advice of sages or philosophers. Or you can trust your own or your friends' experiences. If you feel a foreskin enhances the sexual experience, then don't circumcise your son. But don't be surprised if one day your adult son has his foreskin removed because his sex partner thinks he will be a better partner without it. Your son's sex life will be shaped by his feelings and choices. Or you can go with the odds, but know that the odds are fairly balanced—pro, con, or uncertain—on foreskins.

You can try to make the best decision you can at this time, recognizing that much will depend on unknown factors—your son's modesty or immodesty, his communication skills, his self-discipline, self-control and thoughtfulness, the needs and desires of his partner or partners, and the styles of his future time—and hope you reasoned wisely. Or, you can decide to place your trust in those who believe that leaving your son the way he was created—with a foreskin—will ensure the best sexual experience for him and his partner or partners. Remember that sexual satisfaction—like good dining—is not determined merely by the cells of the penis. It is also, and more importantly, connected to the cells in one's brain, the feelings of one's heart and the spirituality of one's soul.

SECTION THREE

Other issues

CHAPTER NINE

Can a foreskin be restored?

To help you make a fully informed decision, we decided to explore the question of whether or not it is possible to reverse a circumcision—that is, to restore the foreskin. It is a question that has been asked for centuries.

It is hard to imagine a man walking around with a lead fishing weight taped to the skin of his circumcised penis, pulling the skin down in order to stretch it into a foreskin. Other circumcised men try to stretch the remaining skin on the penis by using surgical tape and elastic bands that they wear for up to three years, which is how long it can take to safely stretch the skin—if indeed they have a foreskin remnant to stretch. (The ordeal is sort of like wearing braces to straighten your teeth—it's a long-term hassle, but a man who wants a restored foreskin may be willing to put up with the hassle.) Other men resort to expensive, painful, and not always successful surgery to create a new foreskin.

Whether by surgical or non-surgical methods, the aim is to restore or regenerate the tissue removed by circumcision, and to provide coverage of the glans. All the methods require resolve and patience, and involve discomfort, inconvenience, and sometimes pain.

In a surgical method called foreskin reconstruction, skin from the scrotum (the sac that holds the testicles) is grafted onto the back of the penile shaft. The process can involve a series of surgeries, some risk, and the results are often unsatisfactory. Moreover, the method is costly and medical insurance rarely covers it.

For non-surgical restoration, there is no wizard's formula nor any pharmaceutical available for instant results. The safest and most satisfactory method is through slow tissue stretching or tissue expansion (called "tugging" on the on-line sites dedicated to foreskin restoration). If any penile skin or any of the mucosal lining of the foreskin is left after circumcision, it can be expanded. The remaining skin is pulled down toward the glans, then tension is applied by attaching a weight, or with tape or elastic straps, or with a special "tension restorer device." The amount of tension must be carefully gauged to avoid pain or damage to the tissue.

Tissue stretching can stimulate the growth of new skin, and the new skin will be similar to the lost (original) skin. In time, the new skin can grow to cover the glans. This process can take several years, depending on the amount of skin available to start with, the amount needed, the techniques used, the man's commitment and the characteristics of his body.

Results of the various methods are mixed. Often the new skin looks like a natural foreskin, but lacks some features of the original that cannot be re-created—such as the ridged band inside the tip of the foreskin and the frenulum. The new skin will have nerve cells, but it will rarely be as fully sensitive as a natural foreskin.

Nothing new

Foreskin restoration is almost as old as circumcision. Whenever, in history, the Jewish people faced political or religious persecution, the Seal of the Covenant on the foreskin became a dangerous identifier rather than a valued confirmation, and some men sought ways to conceal it. About 334 BCE, Alexander the Great conquered the lands along the Eastern Mediterranean Sea, home to many Jews. His conquest was not merely military—he and his followers introduced Greek culture, ideals of beauty and health, and popular Greek customs. These included athletic exercises and competitions, in gymnasiums and in public arenas—with the athletes appearing nude. (Women were banned from attending, by the way.) Public bathhouses were favorite gathering places, where many men (especially the wealthy and well-connected) met for companionship, to talk about business and politics, and to gossip—while nude. But to the Greeks, circumcision was a mutilation of the body, and an exposed glans was considered indecent and vulgar.

This social taboo against an exposed glans left circumcised Jewish men in a tight and unpleasant spot—feeling ostracized, uncultured and the subject of crude jokes and satires. Many tried to cover their glans by stretching the skin left after circumcision. This was not difficult as most of the foreskin was still intact. (Remember the original method of Jewish circumcision was to cut only the tip of the foreskin and not remove the entire foreskin.)

In those days, a Jewish man restoring his foreskin was called a mashuk. The process of restoration, or uncircumcising, was known as epispasm, from Greek words meaning, "to draw in." (An ancient and painful method of reversing circumcision was to stretch any remnant of the foreskin, then draw it in, gather it together over the glans, tie it, and apply glue to keep it tightly gathered.)

While a mashuk might have been delighted with his uncircumcision, which allowed him to mix freely with Greeks and Romans, the rabbis were less delighted. In fact, uncircumcision so displeased and angered them that they decided to change the way circumcisions were performed. Thus, about 140 CE, the rabbis ordered that instead of removing only the outer tip of the foreskin (the part that extends beyond the glans), mohels were instructed to cut off and remove the entire foreskin so that a circumcised man could not disguise his Jewish identity.

With the foreskin completely removed, uncircumcision was nearly impossible—except through surgery. And if modern surgical techniques to restore a foreskin are often less than satisfactory, it was unlikely to have been a good option in the second century.

The tragic era

Throughout history Jews were persecuted—for being Jewish, for not converting to Christianity or to Islam, for being different. During the Holocaust, however, a circumcision was often a death sentence. In Europe, during that period, circumcision was not common among non-Jews. Thus, checking for a circumcision was the easiest way to confirm Jewish identity. Jewish males were hunted and forced to strip to reveal the circumcised penis that would mark them as Jews. To prevent detection was nearly impossible, but a few males did find doctors who devised surgical techniques to uncircumcise. While there are no official records—these doctors were working undercover, and at great personal risk—some personal accounts do exist.

Never the real deal

If only a tiny portion of foreskin was removed, as in ancient days, restoration might be relatively straightforward and successful. But when the entire foreskin, including the inner mucosal lining and the frenulum and the ridged band within the tip of the foreskin, is removed, restoring the foreskin is not easy.

Loose foreskins

First, even if a man grows enough skin to cover the glans, the new skin can be too loose. A surgeon can tighten the skin at the tip, but tightening it too much would make it difficult to achieve an erection or to pull the foreskin back over the glans.

No frenulum, no ridged band

Without frenulum tissue, and without the muscle fibers in the ridged band—which can only be restored through surgery—a new foreskin has a tendency not to stay forward.

No mucus

If no foreskin is left, there is no lining tissue left. Since lining tissue contains the mucus-producing cells, it is not possible to restore a mucus-producing ability.

Recently some doctors have begun researching the possibility of regenerating a male's foreskin using the DNA in the person's cells to cause the foreskin to regenerate. This project is in early stages of research.

Currently, we are seeing a movement to persuade parents to leave their newborn sons intact and even to ban routine neonatal circumcision. We are also seeing the formation of groups that offer information (posted on the Internet) about procedures and devices to restore the foreskin—primarily through stretching. There are also ads for products that create a synthetic foreskin, with the aim of protecting the glans from coming in contact with irritants and thereby losing sensitivity. (For more information about reconstruction or restoration, check the websites of UNCIRC, NOCIRC, NOHARMM, D.O.C., and NORM.)

Another (probably controversial) new idea is the suggestion that Jewish law might allow reversing a circumcision because the "mitzvah" is to have a brit milah, but no mention is made of an obligation to *remain* circumcised. This could be an interesting question for rabbis, but is outside the scope of this book.

Advice—whether asked for or not

What we wish to say is: don't go ahead with a circumcision thinking that your son can always have it reversed. While it is possible that he may achieve a semblance of a foreskin, it is more likely that he won't. And the end result—the "semblance" of a foreskin—will never be quite the real deal.

CHAPTER TEN

Whose right is it to make the decision?

Who has the right to decide and the responsibility whether your son is circumcised? You? Or your son (when he is older)?

When we face a complicated decision, it may be tempting, or seem simpler, to follow the traditional path. Historically, parents were considered to have the right to make this decision—and many others—for a son. Jews and Muslims claim fathers have this right because in Genesis 17, God commands Abraham and all the fathers of future generations to circumcise their sons. In Judaism, in the absence of the father, the mother or the community assumes the right to circumcise a male child.

In our contemporary social climate, however, the decision to circumcise and every aspect of circumcision is now questioned and debated—especially health benefits and risks and the importance of pain relief, plus effects on sex, respecting tradition or the cultural norm, and more. However, the most heated debate today centers not on health, sex or religious issues, but on the issue of human rights. And the most vocal in that debate are human rights activists, legal scholars, ethicists and medical associations—while most doctors, circumcisers and religious authorities often retreat from the field.

Most parents who choose to circumcise their sons today are motivated by religious or cultural—rather than medical—reasons. (Although some parents elect to circumcise their sons for potential health benefits.) While it is widely recognized that circumcision is a central tenet of Judaism, honored by Jews since the time of Abraham; and is a ritual observed by Muslims throughout the world, many people are troubled by moral concerns:

- Do parents have the right to circumcise an infant son without his consent?
- Since an infant cannot give consent, does circumcision deny him his basic human rights? (a slight variant or expansion of the first point)
- Does infant circumcision deny a boy his right to bodily integrity and self-determination?
- Is it ethical to remove healthy tissue from an infant?

Some activists state that circumcision surgery infringes on individual autonomy, and is therefore a violation of the infant's rights.

The birth of children's rights

As recently as a hundred years ago, little consideration was given to children's rights. Children had no guaranteed right to education. Children had no recognized right to adequate meals, a home, and medical care. They had no recognized right to be protected from parental abuse or neglect. The only recourse a child had was the ability to run away from home—which many children did.

In the 1920s, a movement for the rights of labor formed. Workers demanded safe working environments and fair pay. Advocates for children began a similar struggle to protect children. Their mission was to ensure that children's basic needs for food, shelter, health care, and education were met. The leaders of this movement were social workers, labor organizers and others dedicated to the welfare of children.

In this first wave of activism, the emphasis was on protecting children. This meant ensuring that the state provided education, limited child labor, created a juvenile court system and took responsibility for children's general well-being.

During the 1960s, the impassioned movements for civil rights, women's rights, gay rights, individual autonomy and personal freedom sparked a second wave of activism for children. The first battle had been directed at achieving "what was good for children"—education, health care, protection from abuse. The new focus was to protect children's individual, personal rights. We could describe this as a shift of attention from needs to rights; from taking care of children to empowering them.

Fathers, mothers and Uncle Sam

In the United States, parents have both the right and the responsibility to make decisions in the best interests of their children. The U.S. Constitution guarantees the free exercise of religion and the separation of state and religion—which is the basic principle by which parents have the right to choose to circumcise a newborn son for religious reasons. Parents have the right to choose to have an infant's disfiguring birthmark removed. They can authorize a life-threatening operation to separate co-joined twins. They have the right—and the obligation—to make medical decisions and, indeed, they may not deny their children any medically necessary treatment, even if their religion or culture forbids it.

Parents have the responsibility for their children and the primary control over the details of their children's upbringing. They can determine their child's religion, and make decisions about their child's schooling. If a parent neglects a child's education, the state can take over the responsibility. If a parent abuses a child, the state can act to remove the child from the parent's custody. However, the state cannot impose a religious view or practices on a child, nor allow a minor child to follow a religion the parents find objectionable. As an example, Jenny was an infant when her Jewish father died. At twelve, Jenny chose to explore her deceased father's religion. Although her mother and stepfather opposed organized religion, they allowed her to attend the local temple and its religious school. But when Jenny declared that she wanted to practice Judaism, her mother and stepfather withdrew her from the school. As an adult, Jenny would be free to practice any religion or none. As a minor, her parents had the right to determine her religion.

Not everyone agrees

> All human beings are born free and equal in dignity and rights. They are endowed with reason and conscience and should act toward one another in a spirit of brotherhood.
>
> – Article 1 of the United Nations
> Universal Declaration of Human Rights.

Certain rights are basic rights, human rights or natural rights. And some people believe that a parent's right to raise a child is so basic it precedes the establishment of government and overrides all civil laws. They believe that government has no right to invade their private lives and tell them how to raise their children.

In contrast, others argue that families exist within the structure of society. Consequently, society has the power, and the right—by law—to regulate families. This reasoning is what protects family members from domestic violence, parental abuse and other threats. By opening the family to public regulation, male dominance over women is weakened. By opening the family to public oversight, parental dominance over children is weakened.

A religious paradox

Despite the commandment to circumcise a son, Judaic tradition provides its own, contradictory ethical argument against circumcision. Jewish law states that it is forbidden to hurt living things. Even necessary pain—such as pain caused when cutting out a tumor—is seen as wrong. This is especially relevant now that we understand infants do register pain, and circumcision pain is severe. Cutting off a natural, healthy body part, even a foreskin, would seem to go against this law forbidding acts that cause pain.

Some Jewish critics of circumcision seek an accommodation, and offer the idea that a carefully considered, rational decision against circumcision can be maintained within Jewish tradition. One Conservative Jewish father, at the Second International Symposium on Circumcision, suggested that the ritual of circumcision "is one of the mistakes Judaism carries within it," and proposed an alternative ceremony which would not include cutting.

Other practices described in the Bible have been condemned, or abandoned. Think about polygamy, slavery, animal sacrifices, purification rites—all left far behind in history. Some Jewish scholars, and many Jews who wish to continue within Jewish tradition, suggest that the current circumcision procedure (which in early times required only a small incision) could be much less invasive and yet satisfy the commandment.

There is irony in the fact that circumcision—originally a religious obligation—gained wide acceptance due to its supporters' claims of health and medical benefits. While a number of these benefits have been largely disproved, for many Jews the ritual survives—perhaps a testament to the significance of the desire for Jewish identity, and perhaps because of a continued belief in health benefits.

International Law

All discussions of medical ethics invariably begin with a reference to the Hippocratic Oath, of the fifth century BCE, which outlined a code of behavior for physicians: "to help the sick. . .[and to] abstain from harming or wronging any man."

After the horrors and abuses of World War II and the Holocaust were revealed, including accounts of doctors performing horrific experiments on human subjects, including infants and children, a clearer and more wide-ranging standard of ethical behavior in medical treatment and research was sought. The Nuremberg Code (1947) made the point that in any medical procedure "voluntary consent of the subject is essential." Later documents, including the 1948 Universal Declaration of Human Rights, the 1959 Declaration of the Rights of the Child, and the United Nations' resolution of the "implementation of the Convention on the Rights of the Child," were directed, in part, at protecting adults and children from all forms of physical or mental abuse.

Opponents of routine infant circumcision take the position that the circumcision procedure (performed without the consent of the child) is abuse. Adding to the arsenal of the anti-circumcision advocates has been the doubt about the medical value of the procedure. Medical organizations in the U. S. and other countries issued statements that seemed to reverse earlier endorsements, or adopted a neutral position. In 1971 the American Academy of Pediatrics stated that there was insufficient medical evidence to support routine circumcision. In 2012, however, after several years of reviewing the findings of over a thousand surveys and studies, the AAP issued a report endorsing elective circumcision. In the report, they advised that parents make the decision, along with advice from their physician. But they also advised that parents be given "nonbiased" information in order to make informed decision (what you are doing by reading this book!).

The website of the Circumcision Reference Library (www.cirp.org) maintains an up-to-date directory of policy statements on routine neonatal circumcision issued by national medical organizations in English-speaking nations. Before the 2012 revised AAP statement, most organizations were consistent in their conclusions. They stated that there were no medical indications for routine, non-therapeutic procedures and officially discouraged them. It will be interesting to see if the AAP's new policy statement—that circumcision does offer potential medical benefits—leads to changes in policy statements by medical organizations of other countries.

Many of the national organizations continue to express concern about the ethical issue of performing non-essential surgery on an infant unable to provide consent. Some specify that both parents consent to the procedure.

That last phrase raises a new issue. If parents disagree on whether to circumcise, should the decision be made by the parent who feels most strongly? Or should the decision be deferred until they reach an agreement?

A legal update

In 2011 an intactivist group in San Francisco proposed a local ballot initiative to ban newborn male circumcision. The initiative failed after a judge ruled that state law prevents local jurisdictions from regulating health care professionals. The initiative was based on the principle of separation of church and state, but the ruling was based on state law. It seems likely that intactivist groups will renew efforts to ban circumcision.

In July 2012, a regional court in Cologne, Germany, issued a ban against elective circumcision as a violation of children's rights. This caused an uproar among the country's large Muslim community and its Jewish community, who viewed it as a denial of their religious freedom. A few state-run hospitals in Austria and Switzerland supported the ban and angry debates erupted in Germany and elsewhere.

Germany's Chancellor Angela Merkel harshly criticized the ban and proposed legislation to overturn it. The legislation was approved, with the stipulations that the circumciser be adequately trained, that effective pain relief be provided, that the parents be advised of risks, and that the child be healthy enough to undergo the procedure. This approval has ensured that elective circumcision will remain legal throughout Germany.

The attempts to ban circumcision have elicited strong protests, especially from Jewish and Muslim groups, and media outlets in Israel and elsewhere. To counter these ban attempts, circumcision advocates note that recent campaigns to circumcise adult men in Africa reduced the spread of AIDS through female to male sexual transmission by an estimated 40 to 60 percent. In addition, the American Academy of Pediatrics' 2012 endorsement of elective infant circumcision for its potential medical benefits has attracted widespread support and media attention.

Back to you

It is an accepted tradition today that parents have the right to determine what is in the best interests of a child—although a government may set limits on parental choices if they are judged contrary to those best interests.

Legally, and by the precepts of many religions and cultures, parents do have the right to choose circumcision for a son. Supporters argue that when circumcision is considered in a cultural and religious context, informed parental consent is enough to provide an ethical base for the procedure. Thus, if you believe that circumcision is in your son's best interests, then you do have the right to circumcise him. But, if you believe that it is in your son's best interest to remain intact and uncircumcised, then you have the right or even the duty, to leave him intact—thus giving him the right to decide for himself. As an adult, he can make his own decision about circumcision.

CHAPTER ELEVEN

Is it moral to have your son circumcised?

At some point in their lives, usually between puberty and maturity, many men devote a certain amount of attention to their penis—judging its size, shape, and overall appearance.

What most don't tend to do, however, is focus on the status of their foreskin and whether it is missing or intact—unless someone teases them in the locker room, or they stumble upon a website condemning circumcision. Or unless they have heard an outspoken radio personality's rant about his circumcision: "I despise it! I despise it! I despise it!" What parent would want to risk that kind of anger over a decision intended to benefit a son?

By now, you have read a lot about circumcision. We have presented the issues and arguments, and facts to help you explore the medical, cultural and sexual considerations that bear on a circumcision decision. We have discussed whose decision it ought to be. These issues are all important. This chapter looks at another important consideration—the ethics of circumcision, and considers these questions:

- Is it right, or moral, to remove a healthy foreskin from a healthy infant?
- As female circumcision may be labeled mutilation, is male circumcision also mutilation?
- And finally, if circumcision is not ethical, should it remain legal, or should it be banned?

Is circumcision harmful?

The starting point for thinking about the morality of circumcision is: does circumcision do harm to the infant? In an earlier chapter, we discussed the importance of safety precautions and the necessity of providing effective pain medication during circumcision. Trusting that these concerns are met, some questions remain: does circumcision do physical harm to the infant? Does it cause unjustifiable pain and trauma? Does it harm his future sexuality? Does it mutilate a part of the body?

Pain and trauma?

Circumcision without pain relief may cause serious trauma. Studies have shown that children not protected by pain relief later react more strongly to the pain of childhood vaccinations, and their responses to other physical pain may be permanently affected. Some psychologists claim it may weaken the mother-infant bonding experience and cause long-term anxiety.

Physical harm?

Clearly, a botched circumcision can cause harm to the penis. For example, a circumcision that removes too much skin can, later, make erections painful or impossible to achieve. In some instances, certain techniques used by very traditional circumcisers can infect an infant with a serious disease such as syphilis or HIV. In cases such as these, one could argue that while circumcision itself may not be wrong, the *method* or *technique* is wrong.

Harmful impact on sex?

Is it right or acceptable to remove sexually sensitive tissue? We discussed the possible physical impact in our chapter about circumcision and sex. But since the sex issue is frequently used both to justify circumcision and to justify leaving a boy intact, we'd like to look at it from a moral perspective.

Attitudes about the morality of circumcision have changed through the centuries, and continue to shift. The philosopher Maimonides, of the Middle Ages, claimed that circumcision dials down a man's lust and is therefore of moral benefit. During the Victorian period, circumcision was credited with curbing masturbation, which was considered a vile habit and the cause of afflictions as varied as tuberculosis, syphilis and insanity. These beliefs have long been abandoned. And have lost moral power. But, in contrast to that reasoning, is it valid to assert that if circumcision has negative effects on sexuality (a debated assertion—see Chapter 8), it is therefore immoral?

Most circumcised men and their partners report satisfactory, good and even fabulous sex. (A recent study reported that the most sexually savvy respondents tended to be circumcised men!) Still, a circumcision removes a foreskin that can provide sensitivity, produce a lubricant, and contribute to sexual stimulation. Thus a case can be made that circumcision can diminish sexual satisfaction for some males and is therefore wrong. On the other hand, intact males are more likely to be constrained by a tight foreskin that interferes with a comfortable erection.

So, a case can be made that circumcision is good for sex, and therefore a morally sound choice.

In reality, it is impossible to predict your son's future sex life—which means it is impossible to judge the rightness or wrongness of circumcision on the basis of the sexual-satisfaction issue. Although—if you decide to circumcise—it is your responsibility to select a competent circumciser. Why? Because a botched or poorly-done circumcision is one of the reasons most frequently cited by those who lament their circumcisions.

Is circumcision a form of mutilation?

> I was circumcised as a baby and ended up with a super-tight circumcision, which has... scarred me for life. I blame my parents.... I cannot understand how an intelligent, free-thinking individual can agree to have a son mutilated for no medical reason.
>
> – Posted on a parenting website.

The common definition of mutilation is "the cutting off, disfigurement, or damage of an essential part or parts of a person or animal." Mutilation is abhorred in the Bible, condemned even before Abraham's Covenant of Circumcision. It has been considered immoral and wrong by most societies throughout history and today. But Jews have been circumcising their sons for thousands of years, and they see circumcision as a mitzvah—both a good deed and a commandment. Muslims have been circumcising their sons since the seventh century. The Muslim circumcision rite is known as Khitan and is also called Tahara, which refers to cleanliness. It is valued as a hygienic measure and as it enables men to follow in the path of the Prophet Mohammed. And in some regions of Africa today, it is seen as a life-saving preventive procedure. For many other people, circumcision is a private, individual choice. For none of these people is there any intent to harm, nor wish to harm or mutilate.

Mistakes

A person unlucky enough to be the victim of a botched circumcision may *feel* mutilated. The way to reduce the risk of a mutilated penis is to choose a medically competent, licensed circumciser. That said, does an accidental cutting off of too little or too much tissue, or cutting off part of or the entire glans, make the act of circumcision wrong? A botched circumcision is often a mistake, a serious and sad mistake. But even tragic mistakes are not mutilations, although the person may feel mutilated. The parents made a decision that they believed was in their son's best interest. Their intent was never to harm, which brings us to an important factor in this debate about the ethics of circumcision.

Intent to harm

Accidental harm may be tragic but is not necessarily immoral, except perhaps, if it was due to neglect or malice. The parents and circumciser who intended good are not to be condemned. In a contrasting scenario, imagine a person is drugged to enable someone to remove one of his kidneys, with the intent of selling it. This is illegal, of course, and terribly wrong, even if the kidney recipient's life is saved. In centuries past, slaves, indentured servants and victims of military conquests were sometimes forcibly circumcised. When the intent was to punish men by circumcising or branding them, the act was immoral and mutilating. When parents decide to have their son circumcised in the belief that it will prevent potential medical problems, or allow him to assimilate into their culture, or to honor a religious obligation, the action is not immoral since the parents' intent is to benefit the son.

Feeling wronged

The righteousness of the intent may not lessen the circumcised son's anger or distress about having been circumcised. He may feel wronged and mutilated.

A person whose jawbone is removed because of a cancerous tumor, or a person whose face is severely burned in a kitchen fire may be seen as disfigured, and may feel mutilated. But there was no intent to mutilate, and no immoral act. In contrast, when a woman loses her nose, mouth or ears because her husband has sprayed her face with acid, she has been mutilated. Her mutilation stirs moral outrage and is morally reprehensible.

When the glans is mutilated because the circumciser did not protect it with a shield, or was too old and had trembling hands, or when an infant dies of a disease contracted from a circumciser using a primitive practice to stem the bleeding, we are morally outraged. When a male's circumcision is too tight or is botched and cannot be surgically corrected, or if the male regrets the loss of his foreskin and is angry that he had no control over a decision about his body, he may feel mutilated. The moral outrage and sense of loss these men may feel are often what we hear and read about on anti-circumcision Internet sites.

Most circumcised men do not voice regrets about being circumcised. Many say they are pleased to be circumcised and pleased that the procedure was performed early. Still, we aim to be unbiased in this book, and we do know that for some males a circumcision seems like a mutilation, especially for those who have learned that a foreskin is not a useless flap of skin. Learning that they have lost the foreskin's sexual sensitivity, its ability to stimulate and to lubricate, makes some men feel mutilated and wronged.

A big difference, and the difference matters

Comparing male to female circumcision may seem reasonable, but if we take a closer look the two practices have little similarity.

Male circumcision

In ancient times, circumcision often consisted of removing only the tip of the foreskin that extended beyond the glans. Modern male circumcisions remove all or practically all the foreskin—with some leaving more skin on the penis (loose circumcision) and others leaving less skin (tight circumcision). The glans is never removed intentionally, although it may be accidentally injured or partially removed.

Female circumcision

In contrast to a male circumcision, a female circumcision often removes the clitoris, which is the equivalent of the male's glans. Specific practices may differ by culture and region. In some, the inner labia may also be removed and even the external vulva may be sewn closed, leaving a tiny opening, sometimes only the size of a straw. These radical circumcisions are often performed without pain relief and often not in a sanitary medical setting. They make urination and menstruation difficult, intercourse painful, and vaginal childbirth risky or impossible.

Perhaps if female circumcision were just a token slice in the hood of the clitoris or elsewhere in the vagina, as a blood sacrifice of sorts (as some describe male infant circumcision), we might regard the practice as part of a cultural heritage, akin to stretching the lower lip with a lip plate. We would not condemn that procedure as we do condemn infibulation—the removal of all female genitalia.

Back to intent

The intent of female circumcision is to reduce or eliminate sexual pleasure—only 50 percent of circumcised women experience orgasm—and to ensure that the woman will remain a virgin until marriage, and be more likely to stay faithful after marriage. And in many of the cultures that practice female circumcision, only circumcised females are likely to marry. Uncircumcised females are likely to remain single and are at risk of being forced into prostitution. As a result, mothers and grandmothers feel compelled to have the girls circumcised, not necessarily as infants, but by the time they reach puberty or the age of marriage, which is often even before puberty.

At times, the intent of male circumcision may have been to reduce lust or masturbation, but it was not intended to eliminate sexual satisfaction or make sexual relations painful or impossible. And, while anti-circs argue that male circumcision removes too much of a man's sexual organ and therefore falls into the category of wrongful mutilation, it is significantly less drastic and devastating than female genital cutting.

For some, male circumcision may be a morally uncertain issue. For some, it is morally unacceptable. Others choose not to circumcise their infants because they believe it to be medically unnecessary. But comparing male circumcision to female circumcision is akin to comparing an ordinary carnivore to someone who tears a limb off a living animal to eat it. To a vegetarian, both may seem wrong, but the person eating a live animal's limb is performing an act that is morally reprehensible.

Our criticism of female genital cutting is not a moral argument to use against neonatal male circumcision. Just as slavery was once tolerated but never moral, female infibulation may be tolerated in certain cultures, but we believe it is universally wrong, even if it has not been universally condemned.

Private versus public issue

Attempts to ban circumcision are not new. In the second century BCE, Antiochus IV, the Seleucid ruler of Judea, imposed severe penalties (sometimes death) on those who performed circumcisions, those who allowed them, and even the circumcised children.

In the first century CE, the Roman emperor Hadrian is said to have banned circumcision within his realm. In 1442, the Roman Catholic Church denounced circumcision. Today, the Church maintains a neutral position toward circumcision. Circumcision was banned in Russia, in 1924, during the Communist regime's attempt to stifle religion. The ban aroused an emotional response from supporters of religious freedom, especially as many believed the ban was motivated by anti-Semitism, and many were alarmed by the brutal methods of enforcement.

In 2010 an activist group proposed a ban on circumcision to the Massachusetts legislature. They stated that circumcision was unnecessary, painful and risky, and was unethical, as the infant was unable to give consent. The proposal failed, but its activist supporters (often referred to as Intactivists—as in "leave the foreskin intact"-ivists) remained optimistic about future efforts. In 2011, a group of California activists proposed a ballot measure to ban circumcision for males under eighteen unless medically necessary. They collected enough signatures to put the measure on the ballot. But the ban was challenged in court by several religious organizations. The judge ruled that such a ban would interfere with the exercise of religious freedom and would (illegally) impose regulations on medical practices. As a follow-up, legislation was introduced to prevent local authorities from prohibiting male circumcision. (Note: In the United States and elsewhere, female circumcision has been successfully banned on the grounds that it is a cultural, not a religious, tradition.) In 2012, the city of Cologne, Germany, banned infant circumcision. This stirred a heated (and sometimes angry) debate. Jewish and Muslim groups protested, stating that circumcision is a private decision and a ban infringes on religious freedom. In December 2012, German Lawmakers ended all uncertainty by voting to protect the right to circumcise.

To understand the debate over whether circumcision should be a private or a public issue, we want to shift the focus to the abortion debate—not because the issue is on the same moral ground, but because the debate about it being a private versus a public issue is similar. Two major, and conflicting, issues in the abortion debate are: (1) a woman's personal right to choose and to maintain her rights over her own body, and (2) the right of an embryo or fetus to develop into a person, with the subsidiary question of when does life begin—at fertilization, during fetal development, or after birth?

Morality, truth, or whatever you want to call it, is not always an absolute. Nor is it necessarily found somewhere in the middle. What is right or wrong may lie on one side or the other depending on an individual situation. In other words, morality depends on each individual situation, not on abortion in general. (Yes, we know that pro-life supporters may disagree, because many believe abortion is wrong, regardless of the situation.) For pro-choice advocates, this means that a woman's right to a choice may be greater if she was impregnated by rape or incest than if she was careless about birth control.

We know well that an abortion discussion can take up an entire book, and it is not the topic here. But there is some relevance to the ethics of circumcision, and whether circumcision should be legally banned as a form of mutilation. The position we support is that we believe that circumcision should not be banned, even though individuals, personally, may believe it is wrong. However it can, like abortion, be subject to medical regulation—such as requiring circumcisers to have medical training or be licensed, and allowed to use only medically sound circumcision techniques.

Many medical organizations have stated positions on the issue. But the stand they take is not that circumcision should be banned, but rather that it is not medically necessary despite its potential medical benefits, and that parents should be given full information about the possible benefits and risks. They do not regard infant circumcision as mutilation, as female circumcision is often described today. We believe infant circumcision is your private choice, not the government's choice, and our goal has been to provide the information so you can make an informed, rational choice. That said, if you decide it is wrong, or a mutilation, don't do it.

Now to you and your decision

We believe that parents who choose to circumcise a son and the circumcisers they select are acting with good intentions. And, we have learned, most botched circumcisions and too-tight circumcisions are unfortunate occurrences, and most can be surgically corrected. What is more difficult—even impossible—to correct, is the way a man may feel about having been circumcised as an infant for non-medical reasons. So here are our recommendations:

Minimize the risks of a botched or too-tight circumcision that could cause your son to feel wronged or mutilated. As we have stated, find an experienced, licensed circumciser who uses effective pain relief and a shield to protect the glans.

If you have doubts about the morality of circumcision, consider discussing the issue with an ethicist or a religious adviser, or consider postponing the circumcision. Some adult circumcisions, using new techniques developed for adult men in an African campaign to reduce AIDS transmission, are less daunting and generally safe. General anesthesia is not required. The procedures cause no bleeding or infection, and the risks of a botched circumcision are greatly reduced. These techniques are not yet available in the U.S., but are likely to be by the time your son is a teenager or adult.

If you fear that your son might someday think his circumcision was mutilating, then leave him intact so he can later make the decision himself. Since the age of circumcision varies in Muslim communities, boys may sometimes have a say in the matter. In Jewish law, if a parent doesn't have a son circumcised, the decision shifts to the son when he reaches the age of thirteen, the age of moral responsibility.

Concluding thoughts

Parents who choose to have a son circumcised usually make that decision for righteous reasons—including honoring their religion or cultural traditions, wanting their son to feel comfortable in his society, or with the hope of avoiding potential medical conditions associated with foreskins.

Although most men do not feel mutilated, those who do are far more vocal than those who accept or like their circumcision. Thus, anger or resentment over circumcision is a rising issue. It is also a reason some people seek to ban routine circumcision. With a situation similar to that in the abortion issue, the opposing viewpoints can be debated, and compromise seems unlikely. We believe circumcision should be a private decision and the right to make it protected by the law. If we believed it were mutilation, we would take a totally different stand. And if you do, you may want to take a different stand, also.

How to make your decision

You've read the book and learned about the issues. Perhaps now you know what you want to do. Maybe you knew all along and just needed support. Or maybe you're more confused than ever.

Critics of routine infant circumcision find no reason for it. Supporters counter with reasons to circumcise. There are enough polemics—in books and on the Internet—on both sides. We believe that circumcision can be justified. We also believe leaving an infant intact can be justified. So, remember: there are good reasons for and against circumcision. What is important is finding the right reasons for your son.

Beware of "The List"

People debating any decision often resort to making lists of competing arguments. Here's an illustration of a decision-making list, focused on a simpler issue: "Should we get a cat?"

Reasons to get a cat

1. Cats provide good company.
2. Cats teach children about responsibility.
3. Cats don't have to be walked.
4. Cats curl up in your lap.
5. Cats eat less than dogs.
6. Cats are easy to groom.
7. Cats can be playful.
8. Cats catch mice.
9. Cats don't bark.

Reasons NOT to get a cat

1. Your spouse is so allergic to cats he or she has asthma attacks when near them.
2. Your spouse hates cats.

If you look at each side's arguments, the length of one list may persuade you to let that choice prevail. But length is not the only measure; which list has the stronger, more important and thoughtful arguments?

Here are a few more decision-making suggestions, based on the book, *Smart Choices, A Practical Guide to Making Better Life Decisions,* and we thank one of its authors, Ralph L. Keeney, for advising us on this chapter. These suggestions should help you make a smart decision about circumcising your infant son.

Base a decision on the most compelling arguments

In circumcision, there are so many factors involved that it may seem impossible to make a decision. But now that we—and you—have identified the issues, decide which are most important to you. Focus on that issue or issues, then make your decision.

Eliminate reasons that have lost validity

In earlier times, circumcision had value as it made hygiene easier. While it may be slightly easier to keep a circumcised penis clean, our reliable access to clean water and our greater knowledge of hygiene make care of an intact penis simple. So we suggest canceling out hygiene as a reason to circumcise. Base your decision on another issue—not this one.

A tight or non-retractable foreskin can cause erectile dysfunction, but this condition can also occur in circumcised men, albeit from different causes. Erectile dysfunction can be remedied and treated, in both intact and circumcised men. This factor may be important, but it isn't fully dependent on whether the man is circumcised. So we suggest eliminating this as an issue.

Eliminate the unpredictable

Through surveys and anecdotal evidence we know that many women enjoy or prefer sex with intact men, and that some men circumcised as adults report that sex is better when intact. On the other hand, some men circumcised as adults prefer sex after circumcision. When the subject is oral sex, many women say they prefer a circumcised man. In general, people today are savvier, more open and more experienced about sex than in the past. And remember that many women who were surveyed, even some of the most sexually experienced, did not know if their partner was circumcised or intact!

Regardless of your preference, you cannot know what your son or his partners will prefer. Nor can you know what your son will be like and what the social mores will be like eighteen or twenty-five years from now. With so many unknowns, and so many arguments on each side, we think sex is an unreliable basis for a decision. But—and this is important—if you think it does matter, then let it matter.

Eliminate reasons that may not really matter much

An intact foreskin may enable a boy to masturbate more easily and perhaps more often. And, maybe, because he can masturbate more quickly, he can get back to studying sooner! Seriously, for some parents, masturbation is sinful or disturbing, but circumcision will not really affect whether your son is inclined to masturbate or not. The threats of blindness, brain damage, and other masturbation-caused problems that contributed to making circumcision routine in the past have been shown to be untrue and baseless. And, since it not likely to be a situation a parent can control, we think this issue should not be an important factor in your decision.

Another factor we don't think should carry much weight is whether it is important for boys to look like their dads. We frequently hear parents cite this reason, but as we discussed earlier, boys we interviewed said they rarely noticed or cared whether their penises did or didn't look like those of their dad, their brothers or their cousins. (If, however, you plan to raise your son in a Jewish neighborhood, send him to a Jewish day school and a Jewish camp, and all the men in your family are circumcised, this reason may be important. Ditto if the father cannot be convinced we are right about this.

Eliminate reasons that aren't clear-cut

Circumcision is said to prevent some medical problems of the foreskin, such as phimosis, when the foreskin is too tight. But leaving your son intact will spare him the pain and the possible complications of circumcision, such as bleeding or infection. Each choice involves risks, and you can find experts on each side of most medical issues. We think each side makes valid points, and if you do, too, you will find it hard to make medical issues a deciding factor. If you don't, then go with what you believe. As we have said, you are making the decision.

A reason that should not be ignored

The Jewish issue

Jews as a people are not willing or ready to give up circumcision. For them, circumcision remains important—as a covenant and as a commitment to their Jewish heritage. So respect this feeling, but remember that circumcision is not what makes a man Jewish. While you may defy tradition by not circumcising your son, you will not rob him of his Judaism or his right to be part of the Jewish people. That is clear, even if some people don't know it. But since most Jewish men are circumcised, a circumcision will make your son look Jewish—when he is naked. If your son has a Jewish parent, gets a Jewish education and lives a Jewish life, he will be Jewish—with a foreskin or without one. Even without the education and life choices, he may still be Jewish.

The Muslim issue

In Islam, males are expected to be circumcised, to follow the way of life of the Prophet Mohammed, and as a rite of passage and a symbol of being a member of the Islamic community.

Improving on nature versus leaving nature alone

Some people elect to leave their sons intact because they believe that foreskins are natural, and natural is good. Some people think nature can be improved upon—through plastic surgery, implants, tattoos, hair dye, eyebrow tweezing, shaving or whatever. Leaving things as they are or choosing to circumcise—it's your call here, which may depend on how you think about the next issue.

The right to make the decision

You may believe it is your responsibility, or right, to decide about circumcision. Or you may believe a boy has a right to a foreskin, and that circumcision should be his decision to make, when he grows up. You can leave the decision for him to make later, knowing that he will be less likely to be circumcised, that it will cost more, possibly hurt more and involve complications, and be slower to heal. On the other hand, with some new techniques being developed, an adult circumcision is likely to be less costly than it is now, be bloodless, painless, and have fewer, if any, complications.

If you make the decision now, your son may later feel relieved at not having to deal with the decision. Or, he may feel resentful and angry that he was not given the chance to make his own decision. Impossible to know.

Get the facts right

Both circs and anti-circs will gladly supply you with statistics: statistics about the medical risks or benefits, statistics on sexual satisfaction or dissatisfaction, statistics to refute or substantiate the risk of penile cancer, and many others. When you consider this data, especially that relating to medical risks, search for the most careful and respected sources, and the most unbiased studies, and learn not to be misled by the statistics. Read carefully to see that the statistics are comparing apples to apples, and that they are relevant. Some reports, for example, state that the risk of acquiring HIV/AIDS if you aren't circumcised is over 50 percent. But that statistic is based on studies in Africa, where there are many variables, and much higher risks of acquiring HIV from a sex partner. Men here face lower risks, unless they are gay (and then circumcision won't help) or are needle-sharing drug-users (and circumcision won't help them either).

Look at risk statistics from both sides

The medical risk of a complication (usually minor) from circumcision ranges from 0.1 percent to 8 percent. That's one side of the statistic. The other side is that the chance of a uneventful circumcision is 92 to 99.9 percent.

If intact, the lifetime risk of a tight foreskin or a urinary tract infection is about 10 percent. The other side of this statistic is that the chance of never having a problem (which is usually minor and treatable) with a foreskin is 90 percent. That statistic improves with good hygiene, good medical care and good habits.

Don't give dramatic events more weight than they deserve

Of course we all are influenced and upset by a distressing outcome—such as a serious hemorrhage or an unsightly circumcision. Remember that such complications are exceedingly rare, and that finding a trained, competent circumciser greatly reduces all risks. And, if you hear of a case in which part of a boy's glans was accidentally sliced off, check the facts before concluding that circumcision is extremely risky. A particular circumciser may be the real risk!

Before your final decision, here are a few things to think about

Are you going to decide by intuition or with logic?

When you need a split-second decision, a gut reaction may be necessary. Smash into the deer dashing across the road or veer into the oncoming car in the opposite lane? An instant reflex is your only guide.

Circumcise the baby or leave him intact? Gut feeling or logic—what should you do? Circumcision isn't a crisis situation, therefore you have time to think. Know who you are. If you tend to make snap decisions, slow down and learn as much as possible about circumcision. Read and think, talk to others, yet also consider your emotional reactions. Then make your decision. If you tend to be rational, be rational about this decision, too.

Consider your tolerance for risk

One reason you may have difficulty deciding is possibly a low tolerance for risk. (Both authors understand, as we each have exceedingly low risk-tolerance.) Weigh the risks of circumcision versus the potential benefits or reasons to circumcise. Ask yourself this: Which could you tolerate better: Your son's anger at not being able to decide about circumcision himself, or his future partner's disappointment about the state of your son's penis? The risk of his not being "Jewish-enough" in the eyes of his grandparents or the risk of feeling that you made a mistake?

Perhaps your partner or spouse, or a good friend can help by giving you the emotional support and reassurance you need to make a decision and carry it through. Instinct and emotions also have a role to play in decision-making.

Prioritize the people involved in the decision

We believe that your first priority is to your son, and your second priority is to you and your partner, to do what you can agree is best. Being a parent allows you to make decisions for your infant, but it doesn't entitle you to make selfish decisions. Thus, if you believe your son should remain intact but you feel uneasy announcing the decision to your or your partner's family, leave him intact and deal with your unease. As a parent, you will likely face worse moments in the years ahead.

Many parents circumcise their sons in order to please their own parents, especially if they are circumcising for religious or cultural reasons. The wishes, feelings and advice of your parents, grandparents, family members and friends may factor into your decision, but the ultimate decision should be what you think is right for your son. Honoring one's parents and treating them with respect is a religious commandment and a virtue. However, we believe (although some may disagree with us) that you have a duty as a parent to put your son's interests first. If you believe it is to your son's benefit to remain intact, or you have strong feelings that you want him to remain intact, then act on those feelings. Your child will become part of his family, and his grandparents will love and adore him. His penis is your concern more than their concern. When he is toddling around and hopping in their laps for a hug and a story, his penis won't be an issue.

The grandparents and great-grandparents of this expected child may want to tell you how they feel about circumcision. Should their feelings and opinions count? With empathy, gratitude for their concern, and perhaps some humor, reassure them that your son will be Jewish or Muslim, even if he has a foreskin. It might help to ask a cleric to reassure them (or give them this book). But perhaps you think family members care a lot about circumcision, and in reality they don't. Or you think they won't care and find out that they do! Advice here: Ask them. Respect them. And do what you think is best for your son.

Speaking of priorities, what if the parents disagree?

When parents disagree on circumcision, a female may defer to a male—thinking he knows more about foreskins and penises. Maybe he does, about sexual and hygiene issues. But given the complexity and importance of the issue, a male should not automatically get to decide just because he has a penis. The best solution is a heartfelt, honest discussion.

The decision to circumcise, alas, can be more difficult in an interfaith family. If a couple cannot agree, the parent whose religion or culture supports circumcision doesn't necessarily deserve the right to decide alone. In families with same-sex parents, whether interfaith or not, open discussion is essential. Both parents should be comfortable with the circumcision decision.

A parent may feel he or she has not fulfilled the biblical commandment to circumcise. In a Jewish family, as we have said, a child who is raised as a Jew, is Jewish. Among more traditional Jews and in Israel, having a non-Jewish mother and no circumcision may require a boy to convert, but that is always an option and nothing to lose sleep over. Circumcision is an obligation in most Islamic teachings—with exceptions for males with medical problems.

If you *still* can't decide

Ask someone to play devil's advocate and argue against you

If you lean toward circumcision, defend the opposite position. If you lean toward leaving your son intact, defend circumcision. If you are uncomfortable attacking the opposing position, perhaps your true feelings are being revealed. If you are comfortable arguing either side, the issue may not be vital to you. You may be comfortable with either decision.

Build those counter-arguments with yourself

If you can't find someone to debate you, debate yourself. This may easier to do on paper, or during a walk in the woods or around the block.

The "What-if" challenge

Instead of a debate, take the following test. We include hypothetical situations and real-life examples.

QUESTION

What if just after birth, a hospital staff member mistakenly whisks off your son for a routine circumcision? Would you be upset? Or would you be relieved that the circumcision took place and you didn't have to make a decision?

QUESTION

What if you can't find a certified, experienced circumciser or physician and therefore leave your son intact? Would you feel relieved? Or cheated? The answer will tell you a lot about how you feel.

QUESTION

What if all the families in your community circumcise their sons? Would you wish you lived elsewhere? Or would you be relieved?

QUESTION

What if it was illegal, or politically dangerous, to circumcise your son, as it has been at times in history? Would you think, "I'm glad I don't have to have him circumcised." Or, "I'll find a way around this."

Advice from all quarters

It is helpful to expose yourself to conflicting opinions and arguments, especially if you are leaning one way but wish to be open-minded. On the other hand, it helps to be cautious about advice from well-meaning family, friends and others who may not understand the issues as thoroughly as you do (especially after reading this book and perhaps doing other research).

Ask the right people for advice

A nurse-midwife or a physician may understand the role of the foreskin and know how to do a circumcision but not fully appreciate the religious or cultural importance of circumcision. Their advice is useful, but you have your own values to consider.

Beware of bias

We have come across many advocacy organizations, websites and experts ready to weigh in with advice—some pro-circ, others anti-circ. You can collect (a lot of) information from these sources, but keep in mind that while they may mean well, they may not be impartial. Some may stridently, or unfairly, work to convince you that their position is the correct and necessary one. We believe that only you can make the right decision for you and your family.

When you are truly perplexed

In ethics and in law, when a difficult issue comes up, scholars and experts often write opinion pieces or interpretations for a publication compiled to present all sides of the issue—majority and minority opinions, and even outliers' dissents. We hope that this book will serve a similar purpose as we tried to present a full range of views on all the issues of circumcision. (And we certainly did a lot of research and thinking, in that effort.)

Most expectant parents have taken circumcision for granted, which is why pregnancy and parenting books devote little space to the subject. But with this issue, it is important to not just accept a popular opinion, without thinking. We believe you need to look at the issues, weigh the choices, decide what matters to you and reach a thoughtful decision. If the minority opinion (which in the U.S. is usually to leave your son intact) makes sense to you and your partner, then go against the majority—but only after you investigate and understand why it is the majority opinion.

The best advice we can offer

First, decide. Decide to circumcise your son *only* if you are sure it is the right thing to do. If you are waffling, wait. If you and your partner cannot agree, wait. If you can't decide, don't decide (meaning, wait). But don't let someone else decide for you.

Uncertainties are part of life

You cannot know for certain how you or your son will feel about your decision in the future. For example, you may regret your decision to circumcise if next year's studies show circumcision offers fewer medical benefits, or if medical advances (such as a new vaccine) eliminate some reasons for circumcision. Or if (and this is unlikely) Reform Judaism and other liberal branches of Judaism abandon circumcision. On the other hand, leaving your son intact may lead to regrets if a new disease that attacks foreskin tissues appears. After all, who in the 1960s would have anticipated HIV in the 1980s?

To put this issue and your decision to rest, remember that carefully thought-out, wise decisions are more likely to lead to good outcomes, but unfortunately, life is not always predictable.

Make the smartest decision that is possible to make now, and make it, preferably, before your son is born. If you decide to have him circumcised, make the smartest choices for when, where, and who is going to perform the circumcision. If you decide to leave him intact, remember the importance of foreskin hygiene (since parents are often the caregivers during the infant's first year, when most UTI's occur) and teach him the importance of hygiene, too. If a problem arises, deal with the problem but don't punish yourself for making what was a smart decision at the time.

You've read this book and perhaps done other research. Maybe you've discussed the issue with people whose opinions you respect. Decide which issues are important to you and the other parent. Take into account your tolerance for risk. Take time for both emotional and intellectual reflection. Again, try to make the decision well before the infant is expected, even if you don't know the gender. Many parents become overwhelmed by childbirth and the reality of becoming parents. Some say they felt pressured into making a decision, and sometimes made a decision they regret. But if you prepare for the child's arrival with the research, the analysis, the self-appraisal and the discussions, you are ready to make a decision. Accept that you are making the smartest decision for your child at this time in your life and in his. Why? Because that is all that is humanly possible for you to do.

OTHER RESOURCES

Books

Glick, Leonard B. *Marked in Your Flesh: Circumcision from Ancient Judea to Modern America.* New York: Oxford University Press, 2005. An ambitious and fascinating study, ranging through religious, medical, social and cultural history.

Goldman, Ronald, Ph.D. *Circumcision, the Hidden Trauma: How an American Cultural Practice Affects Infants and Ultimately Us All.* New York: Vanguard Publications, 1997. A fervent opponent of circumcision's views of the issue.

Gollaher, David L. *Circumcision: A History of the World's Most Controversial Surgery.* New York: Basic Books, 2000. A clear, detailed and intriguing study, by a historian of medicine.

Hammond, John S., Keeney, Ralph L., Raiffa, Howard. *Smart Choices: A Practical Guide to Making Better Decisions.* Boston: Harvard Business School Press, 1999.

Schoen, Ed, MD. *On Circumcision.* Berkeley, RDR Books, 2005. This often-cited one-sided short book argues forcefully for the benefits of circumcision, while dismissing critics and conflicting opinions.

Internet Sites

www.thecircumcisiondecision.com

www.circumcision.org
The website of the Circumcision Resource Center, focused on the controversial aspects of circumcision.

www.circumstitions.com
A website devoted to a review of the arguments against circumcision.

www.cirp.org
This website sponsors the "Circumcision Information and Resource Pages." an Internet resource that provides information about all aspects of circumcision. It includes The Circumcision Reference Library, with technical material, medical and historical articles, and statistics, and The Circumcision Information Pages, directed at parents and educators. The site includes links to information on the rights of children, and on religious and other issues.

www.doctorsopposingcircumcision.org

www.JewishCircumcision.org
A lively discussion of Jewish circumcision, especially for parents in an interfaith marriage.

www.malecircumcision.org
A collaborative global resource center on male circumcision for HIV prevention, sponsored by WHO, UNAIDS, AVAC, FHI, and other organizations.

www.urj.org
The website of the Union for Reform Judaism.

www.MayoClinic.com.
A respected source for medical information.

Organizations

The websites of the organizations listed here provide access to their most recent position papers relating to circumcision, and reports on current research studies and circumcision statistics.

www.aafp.org
American Academy of Family Physicians

www.aap.org
American Academy of Pediatrics

www.ama-assn.org
The American Medical Association

www.auanet.org
The American Urological Association

INDEX

About the Authors

Susan Terkel is the author of numerous nonfiction books about medical and social issues, including *Feeling Safe, Feeling Strong* (one of the earliest books about child sexual abuse) and *Finding Your Way,* a book that explains ethics for teens. Her book, *People Power* was on the American Bookseller Association's "Pick of the List," and *Ethics* was selected as a Hungry Mind Review's "Editor's Choice," and recommended reading by Parents Magazine. *Colonial American Medicine* was selected for Science Books and Film's "Best Children's Books" list. She has written two books about drug policy: the first earned starred reviews; the second was selected for the American Library Association's "100 Books a College-Bound Student Should Read." Recently she coauthored *Small Change,* which was selected as a finalist for Books for a Better Life Award, and featured in USA Today.

Ms. Terkel is a graduate of Cornell University, where she studied Child Development and Family Relationships. She also studied Social Work at Case Western Reserve University. In addition to writing, she is an artist, wife, mother, grandmother and schmoozer.

Lorna Greenberg is a long-time book editor. She has originated and directed a wide range of projects, including books on brain damage, a teen health dictionary, kids and guns, women in the Middle East, a study of creativity, a history of jazz, and numerous biographies of historical figures. She is the author of *AIDS: How It Works in the Body,* which was selected for Science Books and Film's "Best Children's Books" list. She coauthored *Digging into the Past: Pioneers of Archeology* and coauthored *The Circumcision Decision* with Susan Terkel, after editing a number of her previous books.

After graduating from the University of Rochester, Ms. Greenberg earned an M.A. from New York University's Graduate Institute of Book Publishing. She is a wife, mother, and grandmother. She has worked for numerous publishers, and edited hundreds of books. She works as a freelance editor, writer and consultant, specializing in nonfiction.

The Circumcision Decision: An Unbiased Guide for Parents is available at special discounts for bulk purchases in the U.S. by physicians, midwives, birth attendants, birth educators and others.

For more information,
please visit our website or email us at:
www.theCircumcisionDecision.com
info@carrotseedpublishing.com

www.ingramcontent.com/pod-product-compliance
Lightning Source LLC
LaVergne TN
LVHW100730061126
851857LV00011B/472
9780983411574